BEBE

FINDING LOVE

Thor Wesenlund

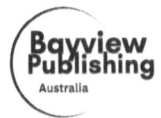

Bayview Publishing Qld

Book Cover by Bayview Studios using Canva

Illustrations by Bayview Studios

Edition 1 2025

ISBN Print 978-1-7641315-0-6

ISBN eBook 978-1-764131-1-3

Dedication

This book is dedicated to all those angels who serve the medical and spiritual needs of people in remote areas around the world regardless of race religion and often in times of conflict and disaster.

Contents

CHAPTER 1

New Beginnings

RENEWAL

I t was late afternoon as the sun was cast long shadows over the endless straight road making it difficult for Bev Anderson as she approached the outskirts of the small town that was to become her. home for who knows how long. Still suffering the pain from her experiences in the city and the recent death of her mother which tipped her into depression.

It was her friend Mary, a fellow nurse from her training days, who helped her and helped steer her toward a new start. It would be a difficult transition from a highly trained nurse with skills in midwifery and trauma and as a theatre nurse in a major public hospital to her new role as an aero paramedic. Still uncertain about the decision she realised there was little left for her in the city.

Her work had been everything to her and nursing was all she ever wanted to do. Concentration on career had left little room in her life for anything else and had cost her relationships along the way.

With her long legs and nice figure, she often stood out from the crowd. In her professional life she was tipped to move to an administrator role, which would be quite an achievement for a 36-year-old.

Unfortunately, that was not to be and her whole life was to be turned upside down after an unfortunate affair with a married surgeon whose well-connected, vindictive wife made life hell. Unable to get any work within the medical field, Bev had taken any job she could find, winding up with menial jobs that barely paid her and her mother's mounting medical expenses. She sold many things, including her expensive car, to cover expenses and now drove an old used one with doubtful reliability her friend Mary had graciously given her.

She was pleased it had gotten her this far and she hoped it would not be needed in her new life. She was tired after the endless hours of driving in this desert-like environment with its straight mesmerizing roads. Looking at the landscape, she was not sure if she had made the right decision but as Mary had said it was a chance for her to renew her spirit and still work in the medical field helping people.

As the small town came into sight down the endless straight road. There was a bang, and the car jumped and swerved off to the side of the road. Had she fallen asleep and lost control and hit someone. The fear mounted in her as she got out of the car and looked around but there was nothing to be seen except a dent on the bonnet and the grill. The setting sun made it difficult to see as she looked around the car for further damage but there was nothing obvious.

Looking back along the road to see if any parts had fallen off, she noticed a brown animal wriggling on the road. Her nurse instincts cut in as she went back to see what it was.

A small kangaroo wandered into her path and been hit. It didn't look too badly hurt so she decided to pick it up and see if she could find a vet or someone to help in town. She was booked into a local motel but it's not likely they would welcome her travelling companion into their rooms she thought.

A few minutes later she pulled into a small service station that appeared to be closing and, catching the attendant's attention, she asked if there was a vet in town who could help her injured furry friend. Pointing down the main road he said

"The Vet might still be there or you can use the number on my window if it's an emergency."

Copying down the number and thanking the attendant she drove off in the direction shown and found the cottage with the Vet sign outside. Knocking on the door she saw a curtain pulled open and face appear. Moments later the door opened.

"Can I help you.

Explaining the situation, she helped the tall young man carry the struggling animal inside,

"I'm awfully sorry for disturbing you up as you appear to be closed." She said noticing his care for the wounded animal as he sedated it and inspected the legs.

"No worries, ma'am" he said placing the animal in a cage and removing his latex gloves and holding out his hand.

"I'm Sam and he's a small eastern grey and it looks like there is no major damage. He will be groggy from the mild sedative I gave him and we will keep him that way till the morning with the drip until I can Xray him for any breakages."

Bev was struck by the gentleness of the man and the way he talked to the animal as if it were a human.

"How many times do I have to tell you guys to stay off the roads, you just don't listen, and you know how reckless these tourists are" he said to the roo winking at Bev.

"Sorry, I'm Bev and I'm moving here to work for AeroMed as a paramedic."

"So, what did you do wrong Bev, apart from running down the natives on arrival." A broad smile crossing his face.

Bev blushed as if this man knew of her past and what hurt she was still feeling. Sensing the hurt in her eyes Sam held out a hand,

"Pleased to meet you Bev, cup of coffee?"

The cup of coffee turned into dinner and late into the evening as they chatted back and forth. Sam looked at his watch and said,

"Have you got somewhere to stay tonight?

"Yes, I'm booked into the Golden Way motel wherever that is."

Sam frowned,

"it's past 8pm and you won't be able to get in there tonight as they close at 8pm. Tell you what, stay here in my ready room, there's a camp bed out there which is reasonably comfortable, and I will see you in the morning to check on our patient."

"I can't do that where will you sleep?" she replied.

"I don't live here, I have a place on the outskirts so you're welcome to stay and keep an eye on the patients for me, there's your roo, a kelpie and parrot and the piglet in the hospital, don't talk to the parrot though, he swears a lot", says Sam grinning.

Bev was so tired from the long drive in her old car and the emotional arrival in town she gladly accepted and put her car in the front driveway as Sam waved goodbye and drove off. It wasn't long before sleep overtook her, and she fell fast asleep to the sounds of the Kelpie snoring and the parrot telling him to F off.

She was still asleep when a young woman woke her with a cup of tea and asked her how she slept. Somewhat dazed and still sleepy she took the tea and nodded, smiling at the young woman standing in front of her.

"I'm Trish, the vet's assistant I was told you brought in a kangaroo last night, so when you're ready we can go and prep it for Xray." she said.

Bev, now wide awake says "Ok but I'm a nurse not a vet or vet assistant so I don't know what to do with animals".

Trish, smiling at Bev, puts a hand on her shoulder.

"So am I Bev, we just have different patients, and Sam tells me you're going to be a paramedic with AeroMed. If that's the case you will find yourself looking after animals and humans, so come with me and I will give you some scrubs and we will get him prepped. Sam is not far away."

Bev reasoned that Trish must be his wife or girlfriend as they seemed quite close when he arrived. In the interim Bev had helped Trish prepare the roo for the Xray by cleaning his fur and giving him a mild sedation. Sam arrived and went straight to work on the roo.

"You will be pleased to know that there are no bones broken and he is just a little bruised. We will keep him here for a few hours and then find somewhere to release him". said Sam smiling.

Bev jumped in quickly asking if she could release him as she felt responsible for his being here.

"Sure, I will give you a call when he is back to normal. Meanwhile do you want a cockatoo? His owner has fled the scene leaving him here to tell everyone to F off. Maybe you could convince your new boss Steve to take him for a receptionist.

Maybe I could interest you in a 2-legged piglet. with training wheels"

They both laughed but the thought of a swearing cockatoo but a 2-legged piglet might suit as a companion when she got her own accommodation.

Trish came inside after looking at the front of Bev's car.

"Sorry Bev but that car of yours isn't going anywhere. Looks like the radiator was damaged in the accident. Best leave it here and I will give Ernie a call to see if he can patch it. You can use my ute to get to town and work and we can cat up later" says Trish tossing her keys to Bev.

Saying goodbye to Sam and Trish for the overnight accommodation she decided to go straight to AeroMed and check in. Making a promise to herself to follow up on Sam who she found attractive, but she did not want to cut some else's grass if he and Trish were an item.

She found her way to the airfield by following the signs and pulled into a parking lot. The building was an impressive 3-storey thing painted in dull green army colours with large hangar buildings on each side and a framed glass tower on top. Strolling into reception the older lady at reception looked up from her desk.

"You must be Bev, How's the roo?"

Bev was taken aback at this knowledge, but the lady just smiled.

"It's a small-town, you'll get used to the bush telegraph. Steve is waiting for you and he doesn't want that rude cockatoo." Motioning toward a set of stairs that led up. Bev paused.

"How do you know about that she asks?"

"Trish is my daughter, welcome to AeroMed Bev, off you go, don't keep the boss waiting on your first day," a broad smile crossed her face.

Bev went upstairs to meet her new boss Steve and turn a new page in her life. Later that first day Sam rang and asked if she would like to come for a drink before releasing the roo. Sensing an opportunity to explore that relationship she readily agreed and went back to reading the textbooks and journals Steve had given her.

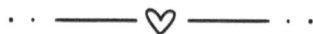

Love is in the air

After dropping her stuff at the motel and putting on her best dress, doing her makeup and wishing she had time to fix her hair she made the best of her assets and headed into town and pulling up in front of the Town and Country pub. Walking in she noticed the chatter stopped and she felt a little vulnerable and paranoid as though the locals knew some of her background and were judging her.

Sam waved from the end of the bar and the chatter continued but the stare followed her as she walked past the line of bar drinkers and into a small lounge. Sam waved to her seat commenting on her attire Sam said.

"The roo will be most impressed that you have dressed for the occasion. Don't mind the guys in the bar, they're harmless and don't see too many beautiful women in dresses around here. I guess you made their day. What are you drinking beautiful lady?"

Bev blushed and asked for a gin and tonic whilst secretly hoping the dashing Vet might be a starter in the romance stakes tonight. After a couple of drinks and more chatting it was clear to Bev that Trish was just his assistant and yes, she had trained as a nurse but preferred working with animals. Bev's interest grew with every word, and she felt this could go somewhere or was it too quick like many of her other romances that fizzled out as quickly as they started.

The meal was basic but enjoyable and they swapped notes on their professional background. Sam had come from the area so after graduating and sometime in city vet's practices, he decided to return to the area. A local vet was retiring and Sam saw an opportunity to buy out his practice along with a considerable client list for a bargain price.

Knowing there were other vets in the district didn't deter him from building the practice based on his reliability and fair dealings. He also set up online group training for station owners to help them treat minor injuries on their stock and pets. His animal shelter was a big hit with the town's folk who were sick of dumped pets becoming pests.

The more they talked the more Bev became attracted to this handsome man with his sparkling eyes and kind considerate ways. She wondered why he hadn't been scooped up by anyone and why he was single but avoided asking that question as it had implications that could kill a relationship in its early stages.

Wondering what his first move would be she waited patiently for Sam to call the shots. When Sam suggested that they go out to drop the roo off she thought this was the move. She will be alone with this hunk in his car out in the countryside at night. Couldn't be better.

I will just go and use the ladies before we go, she said to Sam who went over to pay the bill. In the ladies Bev checked that she had all her assets in the right places and with a quick dab of perfume she headed out to join Sam at the door.

The trip into the dark, cool night cast a romantic mood over her as she took his arm and walked to the Land Rover parked nearby. Sitting as close as she could to Sam on the journey out, she wondered when he would make his move and how best to react. Will he kiss her gently and work up to some fondling.

The rear of the Land Rover didn't look big enough for a full lay down episode but maybe he has a blanket back there. Her mind wondered to the last time she had sex and with the surgeon in the storeroom and how that was a hurried and urgent affair. She didn't think that Sam was that kind and might prefer to go to her hotel room and be more romantic and less hurried.

The back of her mind was saying who cares, get it on with this hunky guy and enjoy yourself. The other part of her brain was saying don't be a one night stand he is too good to lose for that quick pleasure.

They pulled up near the spot where she had hit the kangaroo and Sam suggested she put on a pair of gumboots he had in the back. With her legs out of the door Sam helped her put the boots on and in the process gently touched her legs.

As a shiver ran down her body Sam noticed instantly.

"Are you cold, I've got a jacket in the back for you."

He said handing her a warm jacket that was 2 sizes too big.

Not wishing to explain that the shiver had nothing to do with being cold she put the jacket around her shoulders and stepped out of the car in her gumboots.

Taking her hand, he held the cage in the other as they walked off into the dark landscape with the little roo moving anxiously in the cage. Sams headband lamp showing the way he spoke with the roo in calming tones.

"Don't worry little guy, you will soon be home with your mates. Watch your step Bev its rough out here but it's roo territory" he said pointing to some droppings.

They found a likely area and Sam opened the cage.

"Ok, say goodbye to him and I hope we don't see you again," he said to the roo as it hopped away.

Still holding her hand, he led the way back to Land Rover. The moments for a kiss seemed to come and go as he helped her with her boots and she shivered again at his touch.

"You are cold best I get you home," he said closing her door and jumping into the driver's seat. On the trip back to town. they chatted about Kangaroos and driving at sunset and kangaroo habits of moving from one place to another at dusk.

As they pulled into the motel parking lot Bev's expectations of passion rose to a high level when he touched her hand gently saying

"you've done your penance for Mr. roo"

Bev readied for the kiss that she was sure was coming, only to find he had gotten out of the car and was heading to her side to open her door. It's not over yet, maybe he is waiting for me to ask him in for a drink she thought.

The car door opened for her and with a gentle peck on her cheek he said good night and promised to see her again as he got back to the driver's seat and drove off.

Standing outside her motel room door, feeling let down and just a little horny, the moment had passed and she figured he was not interested in her despite giving all the signs that he was. Maybe it was her and some sort of stigma that she carried. Depressed and anxious again she went to bed wondering if she would ever be right again and find romance and love.

It would be some time later before Sams passions would be revealed.

CHAPTER 2

---◄O►---

AeroMed Life

SETTLING IN

B ev had settled into her life in this rural community and felt valued for her work with AeroMed and the various missions she had been involved in. She was part of a team and her reputation had grown in the district as one of the best that AeroMed had.

Reflecting on the past months, she sat on the balcony overlooking the airfield enjoying her first coffee of the day and an illicit cigarette. The morning sun cast its increasing shadows over the western end of the airfield. Shining like a beacon on the eastern side, the AeroMed building stood out amongst the small hangars and associated businesses.

The building housed the operations center and accommodation for the duty paramedic and pilot. Once owned by the Airforce, it was given to the local community and a grant enabled AeroMed to renovate the dilapidated old control tower and adjacent service buildings and hangers.

Bev always enjoyed taking in the early morning sun and watching the airstrip come to life. She always wondered how many aspiring Airforce pilots in the past had sat up here watching their colleagues taking off and landing and maybe giving them points.

Her thoughts were interrupted by the operations manager Steve Cumming when he appeared from the operation room.

You're up early Bev, I see you're still smoking, not a good look for a nurse, what happened to the patches?" he says frowning.

"Okay Steve, you got me, and I have been trying to quit."

"You know my thoughts and it's not a good look for one of my best Para's to be smoking when we have a program for it. Give it some thought but I really need you to quit, OK" he says with a stern tone in his voice.

Trying to change the subject,

"It's a beautiful morning Steve, got much on today." She says putting out the cigarette in a cup she kept for that purpose. She realised everyone knew she smoked as they could smell it on her and she realised that Steves stern words meant he was getting serious and she must quit.

The 50+ ex Airforce pilot with a prosthetic leg sat down next to her and stared out across the airfield sipping his cup of tea.

"Not a lot today, but there's a rodeo and horse race up north and they always generate problems, but they have enough medical aid and transport options for any injuries without us getting involved, but you never know".

STEVE CUMMINGS

Steve was fit for his age. The loss of his leg in a crash some years back had not dulled his spirit. He had recently received a new leg that allowed him to run again, and he was working up to the local 10km fun run that raised money for AeroMed and other charities. Steves wife was an AeroMed Paramedic and a great friend to Bev when she first moved to the small country town and guided her through the necessary training as well as the lifestyle changes that come from moving from the city to the country.

It became more than a student relationship, Bev's occasional babysitting duties for their grandkids who lived close by and frequent meals made them her close friends. Alice was a light in a dark tunnel for Bev and she was the only one who knew about the city incidents but never judged. Her hand on your shoulder always made her feel safe.

The path to becoming accredited as an airborne paramedic was not easy. Bev found lots to learn like understanding the relationship with your pilot and his authority as well as safety when conducting remote clinics where there have been problems in the past for nurses and doctors. The doctors in AeroMed tended to be young with minimal experience but imbued with a false sense of authority until gently put in their place by the pilots and paramedics who did much of the work.

Pilots were generally older and very experienced. Some ex-military or airline pilots with thousands of flight hours and highly skilled in remote area flying and the inherent dangers associated with the region and the people that inhabited the vast expanses of the outback.

Bev's pilot for most of the time had been Brad Spence. A stern man in his late 50s who had worked in the islands and done a lot of mine recrewing as well as aerial data and mapping work. He was rumored to have had crop dusting experience, but he never spoke much about his past and tended to keep to himself. New paramedics were often scared of him as he tended to push them but was well known and liked by the communities and others in the region.

He tried his thing on Bev when she first flew with him only to be met with a blunt response and smile which he reciprocated. From then on, they knew each other's strengths and weaknesses and made a great team. Brad figured this was his last fling as a stick and rudder man as he called himself. Bev always felt she would crack Brads' hard outer shell and find out what lay underneath the façade before he retired.

Steve broke Bev's thoughts.

"Coming, let's get the morning briefing done and have a little breakfast." He said moving inside.

Alice had arrived earlier and put on the bacon and eggs for everyone. It was one of those things that she often did that endeared her to everyone.

"Right, you lot, don't be shy, grab a plate and tuck in, Steve and Bev are washing up so make a much mess as you can." says Alice,

"Thanks, my darling wife, I'll remember that the next time your car breaks down." says Steve smiling,

The banter went back and forth as the table of Paramedics, mechanics and pilots enjoyed the breakfast and casual meeting which had a serious purpose as well as breakfast. It may have seemed casual, but Steve was taking everything in. From the Aircraft availability and maintenance activity to the training regime and this week's clinics and who was going to fly them. Later that morning Steve would get everything rolling like a well-oiled machine.

The morning breakfast and priorities discussed; the individuals went their own way.

Nodding to Steve as she descended the stairs Bev said, "I've got the animal lectures today Steve so I will be in the classroom for the next couple of hours if you need me."

It was common for the AeroMed paramedics to be able to understand some basic care to domestic and working animals whilst at clinics and on call outs. The Vet had a unique radio frequency exclusive to AeroMed which allowed the paramedics to discuss certain issues in the field. On occasion he had joined a call out flight to a major event if animals were involved but AeroMed couldn't transport injured animals so he was often left to find his own way back from remote cattle stations where he carried out his work.

Today, Bev led a class of new female paramedics with the local vet, Sam discussing dangerous animals and the identification of stock injuries and advice on basics and when to call for help or advice. Bev knew that Sam would be a hit as he always was with the ladies. Introducing Sam, she could see the look in the young women's eyes.

Sam was a stocky well-built late 30's man with sparkling blue eyes and a kind way that endeared him to his patients and their owners. He had gone to the city to train and gain experience but returned home to the town after the vet had decided to retire.

He was very welcome in the town as a local and had many friends. It was always the same old questions after one of his sessions from the young women asking about his marital status. Bev always just brushed it off and reminded them that there were exam questions about the subject and Sam wasn't coming back so she hoped they had taken in what he said.

The Aviation Community

With the session over, Bev returned to the control center to see if anything had popped up on the call out or clinic list. Bev was down for a clinic with Brad in the far north and had to go on standby for a couple of days, which meant living on the base. Nothing new about that for her as she had done it many times before.

The accommodation was sparse but comfortable and she had time to follow her passion for reading and writing short stories.

The sound of an aero engine starting on the AeroMed ramp area meant that Alice was on her way to a clinic and waved as she boarded the Cessna 420 with her kit bag of stuff and presents for the kids.

"Sounds like the flying school is getting busy," says Steve acknowledging Bev and looking over toward the small tin buildings that housed the flight and parachute training school as Alice's Aircraft taxied out.

The school had a couple of ageing Cessna 150's and a 206 as well as a 310 for twin endorsements. Bev had taken to flying in the AeroMed King Airs and housed a secret ambition to learn how to fly one day. Money and time seemed to be against her, but it was on her bucket list, and she watched and learned on every flight with Brad when she sat up in front of the right-hand seat watching him meticulously go through his routines and checks.

In one of his lighter moments, he explained that his instructors from years ago demanded he touch and explain everything he did and received a gently tap on the hand if he got it wrong. Bev was pleased that he was slowly opening to her and wondered what had hurt him so badly to turn him inwards.

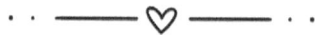

Helicopter Activity

The distant sound of a turbine winding up meant that the Heli flite school at the other end of the airstrip was about to launch one of its bigger choppers, probably the Bell 406 that AeroMed had hired occasionally to fulfill missions that their fixed winged aircraft could not. The owner, Brett Robson, an ex-news chopper pilot was a giant of a man. In his mid-30s he was a singularly unattractive tall man with flaming red hair and paunch with a habit of swearing and telling inappropriate jokes

He often dropped by the AeroMed ops room to check out the talent as he put it. He seemed to be endlessly trying to hit on the female staff of AeroMed to the point where Steve had asked him to refrain and leave on several occasions.

On one occasion someone, locked him in the disused toilet block after luring him away from his amorous attentions toward a new young female paramedic who had recently joined. There was much joy at this amongst the females on the station who took Facebook photos of him peering over the door and begging to be let out. The action turned Bev into a mother figure to the younger nurses knowing she didn't stand for any nonsense. Her and Alice became the go to women for guidance from then on.

Steve let Brett out of the stinky old toilet block after an hour or so and he never came back to the base, preferring to talk with Steve on the phone. He avoided Bev like the plague, and she made a point of making him uncomfortable every time their paths crossed by pointing out that she knew where there was a good dunny (toilet) if he needed one.

Everyone knew about the jibe and what drove it. A picture of him from the Facebook photos in the staff room was always a talking pointed out to new and transferred paramedics with avoidance advice.

Despite this, he was a very skilled helicopter pilot and had done many flood rescues and other work for AeroMed over the years. The rumour was that his wife had left him, and he was on the hunt for a replacement, but his attitude and behavior didn't sit well with the local single women.

He had also had several run ins with local men and had turned up for treatment at the local doctors often. His reputation had not done him any favors in the area, and it was rumored he slept in his hangar office.

Bev felt a bit sorry for him, but his manners would not change, and he was beyond help. One day he announced he was leaving and had sold the business to someone locally. Some months later they heard that after not securing another flying job and working as a cleaner Brett had taken his own life. This added sadness to the station and his picture was taken down in the staff room.

Brett's Replacement

The new chief pilot over at Heli flite was completely different and a joy to work with Andy was ex-Navy and highly experienced having done offshore oil rig and search and rescue work. The first thing he did was to put on a Barbeque for AeroMed and the flying school to introduce himself and the new owner who turned out to be a local station owner and a keen pilot himself.

He brought a new Robinson 4-seater and Switzer to the hanger and Hughes 400 was on order. This gave them considerable training power and attracted a lot of interstate and even overseas students to their facility. This worked well for the owner who also had interest in motels in town and planned to build a bunkhouse off the back of the hangar.

The airfield was becoming busier and there were plans to expand it or move some of the activities like the gliding club and the ultralights to a nearby grass strip. This was of course the sensible thing to do and with some exceptions most agreed, but funding was going to be the problem. Until then there were strict limitations placed on the gliders and the ultralights, which they did not like claiming they were there first, which was correct but times had changed and in the interest of safety they had to move.

In time local and federal funding extended the runway and upgraded the cross runway. New navigation aids were added and the ultralight and gliders were moved to their own area

2 kms away thanks to the generosity of a local farmer gifting some fields and the moving of the hangar sheds from the airport.

CHAPTER 3

———◆◆◆———

Emergency

THE CALL OUT

The day looked like being a slow one and Bev was hoping for an early finish. There was one task she must oversee for the new paramedics that had joined in the previous week. Sam the local Vet regularly ran his dangerous animals and vet care sessions for new starters and as a refresher for those needing it.

It was one of Bev's tasks to oversee these sessions and answer any questions compared to patient care and AeroMed requirements. She also enjoyed seeing Sam and his Kelpie, Kev, who sat patiently at his side until he was needed as a model and hopped up on the table.

For newbies Sam once brought his naughty cockatoo with him, which was such a distraction with his outburst that he was asked not to bring it again and had to repeat the entire session. It seemed that nobody wanted the crested cockatoo despite his efforts. He was even too blue for the pub and his screeches drove everyone mad when the jukebox played certain songs he would screech along with the music.

Sam was popular with the young female nurses who were surprised to find a hunk like him in this remote area. Bev often had to deflect questions about Sam and his marital status answer post session as she just didn't know and her date with him had proved unfulfilling. She always found a way to deflect the questions and let the young women find out for themselves. It was the way of the bush she told them.

The session ran with the group young women focused on Sam with more than intellectual attention. Sam ran through all the dangerous animals that they might meet on their missions, how to find snake and spider bite marks and symptoms. Sam often brought pictures and sometimes examples of reptiles and bite replicas. When he pulled a snake out of a bag it made the newbies sit back a bit but they got the message even though it was a relatively harmless python that many farmers kept around to control rats and mice.

The practical part of the sessions involved Kev on the table whilst Sam showed the newbies how to find the various aspects of animal injury and in particular working dogs like Kev. He explained the importance of working dogs and pets to remote farming folk. He went on to explain the Vet care link they would have in their medipaks and how to contact him for advice.

Many new paramedics from the big hospitals found this all rather strange until it was explained that they might encounter requests to look at all sorts of animals during clinics and this is just part of the obligation here and had a direct bearing on mental health, trust and support for the AeroMed services

Sam was well into his closing remarks and about to answer questions when Steve interrupted motioning Bev from the door to come outside.

"We have a call out; man trapped in machinery at Abercrombie farm. Brads getting the Aircraft sorted. What do you need?"

Without hesitation Bev's years of training and experience came in

"Ok, can you get the amputation kit, jaws of life and spanner and socket set please? I will go change and meet you at the Drug safe. I'm going to need morphine and puffer whistles and can you get the ice chest and bags? Might be good to throw in a body bag as well just in case."

"Ok, I will have the radio frequency plates ready for you and tell Brad I've cleared the airfield for his departure but there is an Aircraft in the zone that's not answering. Probably a glider.

Running down the stairs to the locker room she quickly put on her flight overalls and checked the pockets for the essential pens and pads, tissues and thermometer. Her ready bag was checked as she went to the locked cupboard that kept the dangerous drugs secure. Alice was already there, and the 2 key system was used to open the locker.

"Reckon you're going to need Morphine for this one and perhaps some painkillers and green whistles."

Agreeing they were placed in her flight bag locked section along with sterile needles and scalpels. Arriving at the ramp she noted that Brad had one engine running and the other starting. The ground crew had loaded and stowed the tool kits and Jaws in the special holding locker at the back of the cabin. Steve handed her the Radio frequency cards and helped load the medical kit, while she checked the gurneys and straps and the onboard oxygen and defibrillator.

Shutting the hatches, Bev checked the door locks. Looking back over his shoulder Brad asked if she was ready to go. The thumbs up from Bev saw the Aircraft lurch forward as Bev made her way up to the right-hand seat and strapped in.

"No medico today for this one" says Brad.

"No, it's just you and me, my friend, what's the flight time?"

"It takes about 25 minutes to get to the maintenance area strip. It's going to be tight as the strip is barely long enough for this bird." He says, handing Bev a series of approach plates with aerial photos in the corner as they taxied out to the strip, he explained the problem of weight and balance if they take the patients weight into consideration.

"It's going to be touch and go getting off, but I think I can pull it off if we use the whole threshold area providing it's not a mud hole. Anyway, leave that for me to sort out. I will set comms 3 to the Abercrombie frequency when we reach the cruise altitude and you've got the other frequency info I presume.

Lined up after runup checks Brad guns the two mighty Pratt and Whitney turbo props to take off power. Releasing the breaks the Aircraft charges down the airstrip. Bev has taken a keen interest in flying since she got the job, and Brad encouraged her to understand flight dynamics. Having looked at the weight and balance chart during the taxi she had the numbers and called out.

"Airspeed is alive, V1 and rotate" as the air speed reached the correct point.

"Well done that Lady, right on the money, I might make a pilot of you one of these days" said Brad with a not typical smile on his face.

I wish she thought sitting back and noting the rate of climb and air speed. She was beginning to understand this stuff despite never having flown a Aircraft before. Brad sometimes let her take controls for short periods during longer flights when they reached cruising altitudes, which she really enjoyed.

Reaching Cruising altitude and following Brads radio work, Bev sets the radio frequency to Abercrombie station and contacts the manager. After some back and forth it was clear they had a major problem on their hands. The injured man had fallen and trapped his right hand in the jaws of a header. He was unconscious and they had applied a torniquet but had not released the pressure for some time.

Bev gave orders as to what was needed and gave an estimated time of arrival and their intention to use the maintenance airstrip using details she had from Brad.

Having finished the radio chat, she turned to Brad.

"I think we might be transporting a corpse with us or if you're concerned about the strip length, we might be best to get them to take the body by road."

"Ok, let's see what happens, either way, I'm going to check the strip once you're settled in with the patient."

"Good plan, we will soon know what the answer is." She says.

It wasn't long before the vast expanse of the Abercrombie's 100,000-acre farm was in sight.

"Okay, time to get this bird on the ground. I wish we had the homestead runway instead of this dirt track. Keep an eye out for strays and cattle I'll do a precautionary search (PSL) over the area before landing, so let's know if you see anything out your side."

The Aircraft descended and swung around over the dirt strip. The maintenance building in the distance glinted in the afternoon sun as Brad lined up for an approach.

"Nothing out my side Brad"

"Yep, same here, a couple of dogs that's all".

The landing was precise but brutal with clouds of dust spewing up as the reverse thrust was applied. The strip was very rough, and they bounced down the strip and turned back toward the waiting vehicles.

"Our ground crew aren't going to love me for this one Bev. Hope you brought your fly net" he said touching her arm as they came to a halt, and he wound down the engines."

Unbuckling her harness, she pulled the mesh net which was part of her flight suit over her head and shoulders and put on her radio and body cam harness. A quick hi five and they headed to the back of the Aircraft and opened the doors, setting the proximity alarm as they left.

"Brad, I will go to scene with the medikit. Can you follow up in the ute with the extraction equipment and the mini fridge? Once we see what we are dealing with you can come back for the gurney or the body bag as needs dictate." She says doing a quick radio check and switching on her body camera.

"Okay, Bev, off you go I will be right behind you do another test of your radio on the way in."

This technology was new to Bev when she first joined AEROMED. Unfortunately, a necessity since a nurse was raped and murdered during a solo overnight clinic at a remote station some years back.

Also, the amount of legal action had increased to the extent that paramedics and others needed to be able to fully recall all their actions. The Aircraft was equipped with GPS, flight cameras, voice recording, and panic and proximity alarms to dissuade theft of equipment and drugs stored on board.

This technology also served as a training aid for new recruits where lessons could be learned from the experience of others through the video footage they gathered, especially on major accidents like this one appeared to be.

The Abercrombie Incident

The supervisor ushered her to a quad vehicle and they sped off towards a large shed with several people gathered outside the main door. The crowd parted as they approached the large door and came to a halt. Bev checked her radio with Brad and checked her body camera was running.

As she entered the large equipment shed, she was overwhelmed by the smell and general rubbish strewn all over the place. Noticing Bev's look of disdain, the farm supervisor apologized for the mess explaining they were in mid harvest and things have gotten a bit out of hand.

Nodding and moving in the direction pointed out by the supervisor she made her way over pieces of broken equipment, timber and rotting chickpeas ground in amongst the rubbish. Finally reaching the scene she sees a tall man collapsed amongst the debris with his right hand inside the gate of a header. A younger man is kneeling next to him and comforting the semi-conscious man.

As she moved closer, she noticed the younger man holding a damp rag and bottle of water. The patient's right arm had a torniquet applied and when asked the younger man replied that he had applied it and had moments before released it as he had done on earlier occasions at a proper frequency.

Bev nodded and noted the water in the bottle the younger man was holding looked discolored and dirty. Asking the young man if he has given the victim any of the water, he replied that he had as its all they had.

Taking the situations in Bev noted that the bleeding had stopped but the hand had been badly injured. It was clear the machine was inoperative as the gearbox and engine had been removed. Brad arrived with the tools and the ice bucket and they decided they would need to release the hand by taking the blade assembly apart and then binding the hand before putting it into ice before transport.

Bev got a drip going and asked the supervisor to release the hydraulic pressure on the header, asking why these headers don't have guards fitted? The explanation about time and speed did not convince her about the safety attitudes that she felt were lacking.

The patient stirred a little as she put an oxygen mask on him and there was a look of gratitude in his eyes that she would never forget. While waiting for the hydraulic pressure to be released she did what she could to treat the trapped hand and wipe the man's face and arms with some fresh water.

The supervisor signaled that he had released the hydraulic pressure on the header blades and Brad began the delicate removal of the piece of equipment the was trapping the victim's hand.

Bev noticed the bruise and a black eye on the other side of the man's face. Asking if there was any pain anywhere else, he motioned toward his right leg.

Opening his trouser leg, she saw a large gash down his calf with dried blood down the leg. She did some basic treatment for that wound and motioned Brad to take away the final bit of equipment with the supervisor's help. The hand now free showed a severe cut to the fore fingers at the joints and lacerations to the palm.

"Not as bad as we thought Brad would you pass the ice bucket while we get him up on the gurney".

Her skilled hands quickly had the wound wrapped and a quick shot of morphine helped to solve the victim's pain although he didn't cry out. They are tough these farm workers she thinks, asking Brad and the supervisor to take him to the Aircraft whilst I gather some basic information.

She quickly found out the victim spoke little or no English and most of the farm workers were Spanish speaking Filipinos. The young man who had stood by the victim spoke quite good English and explained he had been a med student prior to working on the farm. When his father died, he had to give it up and find work to help support the family.

Walking out of the shed with the young man he said his name was Armando and the patients name was Alfredo. With regards to how the patient had become trapped in the dormant machine, Armando was sheepish and looked scared. Bev put an arm on his shoulder and told him.

"it's okay to let me know, it won't affect your work here."

"You don't understand, we are illegals and are at the mercy of the big boss who threatens us with expulsion and even detention if we say anything. Alfredo was trying to get us better accommodation and the big boss hit him, and he fell into the machine. The big boss turned the manual release and trapped Alfredo's hand then kicked him and hit him with a piece of wood he threw over there. Please don't tell anyone I said anything. There are 15 adults and 8 children here."

Bev looked at Armando in disbelief.

"Did you say there are children here?"

"Yes, they are in the sheds over there," pointing to a line of run-down dilapidated sheds that had seen better days.

"How old are the kids Armando?"

"They range from 5 to 12. The 10- and 12-year-olds work on the farm moving tarps and cleaning."

"You're kidding"

"No, we all work 12 hours a day, 6 days a week but we get Sundays off."

"So where is the mess hall and washing facilities Armando?"

"There are none Maam, that pile of timber over there is what we must use to cook, heat, wash and patch out sheds. There is only bore water for us and no food prep areas."

Looking at the pile of timber Bev notes that its CCA treated pine from old fences etc.

"You burn this" says Bev looking at Armando.

"Yes, Maam it's all we have."

"Armando, this is treated pine timber waste by the look of it and it will give you serious health effects if you burn this. So do not burn this again. OK"

Armando quickly moves away as the supervisor approaches.

Bev with fire in her eyes give it to the supervisor both barrels.

"I want your name and address if it's not here on the farm. There are some serious issues surrounding this event and you can expect to hear from someone soon. In the meantime, get these people some clean water and proper accommodation. I'm taking this piece of timber with blood on it for testing and this piece for CCA testing."

Looking somewhat sheepish the supervisor backs away as Bev heads to the Aircraft. The patient made secure and given some water and pain killer, it was time to go as Brad fired up the engines.

"I hope we can make it out of here", the patients a bit bigger than I thought but we are still inside the weight and balance limits. says Brad.

Strapping in Bev does a final check of Alfredo and gets a nod as Brad heads to the far end of the strip. Standing on the brakes, Brads gates the throttles and with a knowing wink at Bev, he lets off the brakes and they hurtle down the strip towards a hedge row. Bev closes her eyes as they get closer to the hedge.

Seconds later they are airborne and wheels come up with a reassuring thump.

"That was close, what happened to my V1 calls. I will buy you some new underwear when we get back if that's not too personal" he says smiling.

"Underwear would be most welcome Brad; Perhaps I should get you some too." They both giggle whilst Brad sets a course for the regional airport and ambulance requirements whilst Bev heads back to check on Alfredo.

"I don't think we've heard the last of this one" says Bev.

CHAPTER 4

———◆○◆———

Grateful Patient

Bev's New Name

The Aircraft reached its final waypoint as Brad planned his approach to land. Bev checked on the security of the patient and the equipment as well as logging the gear they had used at Abercrombie station whilst Brad made his usual radio calls and received arrival information.

After a final check on Alfredo Bev sat in the jump seat beside him in preparation for landing. Before strapping in she reassured him, letting him know they would soon be landing, and he would be going to hospital. He seemed to be coping well with the pain, but she gave him a puffer to pull on for the final part of the flight just in case. As she reached over to check his straps and his leg dressings his left hand reached out and touched her gently on her arm.

In a hushed voice he whispered,

"Gracias's angel Mio." His eyes smiling up at her with a look she had seen before from grateful patients. It was that look and the gentle touch that kept her faith in nursing and the help she was able to provide. She did not fully understand his words, but her Spanish speaking mother had encouraged her enough to learn a few words.

"De Nada, your welcome," she replied and stroked his head as she made her way back to the right-hand seat and prepared for landing at the regional airport.

Joining the pattern at the large regional airport, Brad announces that they have another call out to Forest farm after we unload.

"Don't tell me Casey Forest has broken something again? says Bev.

"Correct, the roads are closed that way due to minor flooding and it's too far for our Helo friend to reach. The weather doesn't look too good either so they landed at a local airstrip just to be safe. Their little 175 is not equipped for this sort of weather" says Brad.

"Ok, I'm supposing his mother has him stabilize so it's a transport back to here for him and her?"

"No, we are taking them back to the base and the district hospital. She is hoping Charlie will have finished mustering with the family R44 helicopter and they can stick around until Sean is clear to go back to the farm with them."

"Okay, so what's the plan" says Bev.

"Once we offload the patient, I will go get the fuel truck organised, get a weather briefing and get us some coffee. Then we head off. It's only a short hop but likely to be bumpy with this weather closing in."

"Okay, I better check my pain relief stocks and see if the Ambos can spar any in case it's needed. I will also tidy the place up a bit whilst you're gone."

"That sounds like wifey speak", says Brad smiling.

"Just fly the damn Aircraft smart arse." She retorts giving him the bird and smiling but thinking it is kind of a marriage this AeroMed stuff.

Cleared to land they ran through the checks which included the patient checks and seatbelts, missed approach procedure and other items on the printed cards. Runway in sight, landing checks complete, Brad gently put the King Air onto the ground and taxies to their dedicated emergency stand area near the VIP lounge where they could see an ambulance waiting behind the gate for their arrival.

With the engines shut down Bev unbuckled her seat belt and moved toward the back of the Aircraft to open the double doors. The ambulance guys approached the airport emergency services ramp area with all the yellow markings and signs on the tarmac with their gurney ready for the patient transfer to the ambulance.

"Wait for it, yells Brad. Nobody moves till I say so, remember."

"Yes dad, I remember. It's your party."

"Thank you", says Brad noticing Bev has her tongue poking out.

"Less of the attitude nursey" says Brad smiling broadly as he applies the parking brake and checks the engine run down.

With the 2 wide doors open and the stairs down Bev checked with Brad that it was clear to unload. Bev freed up the gurney stops in preparation for unloading with the Ambo's help it wasn't long before Alfredo was loaded into the waiting ambulance. As he was being loaded, he reached out to Bev motioning for her to come closer and pointing to himself he said.

"Alfredo," then pointed to her with a questioning look that could only mean he wanted to know her name.

Bev motioned to herself and said. "My name is Bev."

That look came over Alfredo's face again as he clutched her hand to his chest with his good hand whilst the ambos waited.

"BEBE mi angel de la misericordia." He said.

Bev was overcome with emotion as she gave him a quick hug with tears in her eyes.

Closing the ambulance door, one of the Ambos who was apparently fluent in Spanish turned to Bev as she finished closing the door.

"You've made quite an impression. he said? 'Bev, my angel of mercy' in case you want to know."

They smiled a knowing smile at each other and the ambo headed to the driver's seat and left with the gate being shut behind them.

Brad had left the Aircraft and was standing behind her the ambulance left.

"The usual Flat white BEBE." He said as he walked away.

Bev smiled at the thought. Perhaps she had a new nickname now.

"Please" she says heading back to the Aircraft to tidy up and secure the 2 large doors ready for the next flight.

She was just finishing the tidying up of the storage area and putting away the extra pain killers the Ambos had given her when a smaller Aircraft pulled up right in front of the King air, blocking its path of departure.

ABER air blockage

The small twin-engine Aircraft had barely shut down when the door swung open and its Captain in full uniform alighted and headed toward the VIP lounge. Wondering what this was all about she noted the pilot glaring at her as he entered the VIP lounge.

A second less resplendent pilot appeared at the top of the stairs and Bev stepped down from the King air with the intent of having a chat and asking them if they were aware that they were parked in an emergency Aircraft only ramp area and blocking their departure.

He was a young pilot who was obviously intimidated by the cocky pilot in command.

Before she could head over the young pilot made his way over to Bev and was apologetic and aware of the breach of regulations and had pointed that out but was overruled by the pilot in command. He couldn't move the Aircraft as the pilot in command had taken the keys. He would need a tug to get it moved. Bev tried to reach Brad but noticed he was already heading towards her with two large coffees in his hand.

"Ok Boss, I've spoken with the other pilot who said he cannot move the aircraft without a tug". Passing her the coffee with the words BEBE scribbled on it.

"Here you go, don't sweat it kiddo it's all in hand. How are you Col. I see your still flying with Mr. Wonderful."

"I'm sorry about this Brad, he refused to listen to me or the tower and he has the keys. I've asked for a tug to get us out of your way but I suspect he will counter that and have me fired." said the young pilot.

"You know where I am if he does and trust me, it would be a better career move to get away from that fool before he kills you or someone else" said Brad climbing the ladder into the King Air

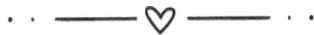

Obnoxious Pilot

It wasn't long before the pilot in command appeared with no shoes on and trousers rolled up and carrying a plastic bag. Glaring at Bev and Brad he yelled out,

"you've not heard the last of this smartarse. You're going to regret your action today."

Bev turned to Brad, looks like you have some history with that creep. What's he talking about??

"That's Nigel Abercrombie, Jack Abercrombie's grandson. I was his flying instructor and washed him out twice before he talked his way around someone and got his licences. He is a creep and a danger in aviation terms."

"So, what's he doing barefoot?" says Bev,

"Well, you know how it is with us old guys and our bladder thing. I had a little accident in the toilet when he tapped me on the shoulder whilst I was midstream and I instinctively turned around and pissed all over his shoes and trousers. He then fell over into the piss on the floor."

"You're kidding me you pissed on a fellow pilot. That's got to be a misdemeanor of some sort."

"Well, it's certainly cost him a charter, look at the passengers at the VIP gate. Notice the attitude? He is finished. The ATC have ordered him to move the Aircraft to a standby ramp and to report to the ATC and airport manager. That guy that has just walked up to the door is the ramp area supervisor and he has the authority to make decisions."

The pair noticed Nigel stepping down and going back to the terminal whilst the ramp guy waved to Brad and closed the door on the small twin as the tug backed up the Aircraft.

"Okay, BEBE, that's the fun for the day, saddle up and let's get down to pick up the young Forest and his mum. You got everything sorted?"

"Sure, have dad and thanks for the new name."

"I think it suits kiddo. I will make sure the word gets around angel BEBE."

They both giggled but knew there was great respect for each other and the job they did as the King air taxied toward the end of the emergency services ramp area.

Looking out towards the far end of the runway and the taxi areas Bev noticed the offending ABER AirAircrafts being towed down to the far end of some hangers.

"Hey Brad, why are they towing the ABER bird down there? I thought they just had to move it. It looks like its heading to the hangar marked Aviation Authority Impound area. Is that serious Brad?"

"You bet, they are in a world of trouble and not for the first time."

"That's a shame, that young pilot seemed quite nice, and apologetic will he be in trouble."

"Unfortunately, I think it's always the flight crew that get the bullet over stuff like this. Don't get me wrong, Colin is a pretty good pilot. I suspect he did most of the flying whilst Nigel took the accolades as usual."

"Nigel was the guy you pissed on asks Bev.

"Yep, he's a piece of work and certainly no friend of mine. When I washed him out on 2 check rides for his Commercial License and he was ropable as was his grandfather Jack Abercrombie who sent young Nigel off to the city with a bucket of money to buy his licences and then set up ABER Air for him to run.

"I'm sure you will meet him and his car dealer mate Alan if you hang around any of the up-market bars in town. He thinks he is god's gift to women and always runs around town in his uniform and wings. Take my advice and avoid him and his mate if you have the misfortune to run into them. Anyway, back to flying this bird. Pre take off checks please Maam."

Checks done and lined up it was off into the late afternoon sky with darkening clouds forming in the distance. Once at cruise altitude, Brad took a last draw on his coffee and flipped the cup into the bag he kept beside him.

"BEBE. I didn't know you spoke Spanish."

"It's a long story, I don't really speak Spanish but my mother came from Columbia, and she would teach me little bits."

"Is that where your dark good looks come from," says Brad, smiling across at Bev as he set the auto pilot.

"Well thank you kind sir, nice to be appreciated, I guess I got a lot of my mother's looks."

"Ok don't let it go to your head BEBE; we've still got work to do although I suspect Amy will have it under control and we will just be the taxi service."

"She was a nurse wasn't she, says Bev."

"Yep, and a damn good one too. She was the district nurse here and we nearly poached her for AeroMed but she went and married Tom Forest and that was that. However, she still runs health clinics near their farm. I'm sure you two will get along, she is a lot like you and can also talk the legs off a table to." Bev gives Brad a gently punch.

"One minute its compliments then insult. No wonder your still single."

"Is that an offer, pretty nurse BEBE," he says smiling.

"Just fly the bloody aircraft hot shot." She replies.

CHAPTER 5

---◆◇◆---

Girlfriend

The Forest Family

The rest of the flight was uneventful, but the weather was on the turn and the cloud base looked like it was descending.

"Okay BEBE, we are going to do an instrument approach into the district strip so I'm going to be a bit busy. Before doing any landing, checks can you go back and check that everything is secure as it's likely to get a bit bumpy."

Agreeing Bev unbuckled her seat belt and headed back checking all the straps and tie downs were tight. Climbing back into the right-hand seat she reports everything secure.

Brad now starts his pre landing and approach protocol chat, so Bev knows what to expect. Following some radio chatter, he begins his checks with Bev helping and enjoying the work even though she was not really needed but Brads rule was if you sat in the right-hand seat you're involved and will take part.

Descending through the clouds it seemed an eternity before the runway came into sight. It wasn't long before they were on the ground and heading to the small terminal building where a couple of figures huddled in the doorway in fading light of day and gathering storm clouds.

Once the engines stopped and the door opened 3 figures approached the hatch with the first one climbing in followed by the lady who must be Amy thought Bev and finally a large man who announced himself Tom. He kissed the women and his son who Bev presumed was Sean and wished them God speed as he stepped down from the hatch and shut the door.

Bev checked the door and made sure everyone was secure as Brad fired up the engines.

AMY

Reaching across the Aircraft Bev held out her hand.

"Hi, I'm Bev, I guess your Amy and this is Sean."

"Yes, but you won't get any sense out of him" pointing to Sean wearing headphones and looking at his tablet.

"He is watching the last Moto GP. Anyway, I've done all that's necessary, so he is comfortable and has had some pain killers. It's not a bad break and should heal as quickly as some of the others he has had."

Bev looking astonished.

"How many has he had?"

"Four, 2 legs and 2 arms. He keeps me current with trauma work that's for sure" says Amy smiling.

"Goodness that's a lot for a young guy his age. Thank God he has you around to fix him up."

"Yes, but he is a fanatical motorcycle rider and hopes to be a professional someday. We have doubts but he has put in the work and appears to be successful in competition so we don't discourage him,"

Little did they know that in years to come he would become champion. But for now, he was just an injured kid and there were papers to be completed once they got airborne.

As Brad got the King Air started, Bev moved back to where Amy was taking Seans Blood pressure and temperature.

"Hey, you're going to put me out of a job lady" says Bev smiling.

"Sorry, force of habit, here's the numbers, he is stable. We might give him another pain puffer in half an hour or so if he feels he needs it but for now he's comfortable."

"Okay, so let's get some paperwork done. Says Bev

Amy hands Bev a folder with neatly written patient information and the forms already completed.

"That was easy, you can come again Amy" says Bev smiling broadly.

"Was that your Husband before."

"Yes, that big lug is my husband, Tom. We planned to fly up to the Base but the weather closed in and our little 175 over there is not up to that sort of flying so we thought it safer to land here and call you guys up, sorry about that." said Amy

The flight was normal if a little bumpy due to the weather. Bev and Amy chatted happily with one eye on Sean as they swapped nursing stories and their backgrounds. The conversation was interrupted by Brad telling them he is on descent for landing and to do the security checks.

"I've got this," says Amy. Referring to Sean and the gurney, Bev checked the back of the cabin and moved back to her seat up front.

The home base airfield came into sight and Brads familiar call for landing checks were made. Looking at Bev as she runs through the checklist's cards Amy comments.

"Gawd, does he make you do that as well," says Amy.

"I certainly do Amy; you remember me trying to get you involved during your trail period with us."

"Oh yes, I do sir. You're still a bloody Tyrant I see".

Brad smiled at himself and pointed at Bev.

"This one is thinking of learning to fly like you did."

Bev turned around and said, "You're a pilot Amy,

"Yes, I did my private license with this tyrant as my instructor. Man, what a job that was. I don't know how you put up with him at work. Thank God he knows how to fly"?

"He's OK, once you know how to manage him. If all else fails, I hit him. Get him to show you the bruises sometime. says Bev They all laugh.

"Ok ladies turning down wind leave me alone and don't hit me during landing please. Captains' orders."

They touched down and taxied to the AeroMed ramp and a waiting Ambulance. Loading Sean into the back of the ambulance one of the Ambos said,

"Hi Amy, what's he done this time?

"It's in the folder, Stan" she says handing over the patient info folder.

Turning back before getting into the ambulance she says to Bev.

"I'm likely to be in town for a couple of days, if you're off tomorrow how's about catching up for coffee and some girl shop stuff, call me in the morning and we will plan something. The ambulance doors shut, and it headed off to town with just its lights on.

Turning to Bev Brad says

"OK BEBE let's get this bird cleaned up and put away so we can go get some rest."

Steve had wandered out to greet them and said.

I hear you have a new name BEBE.

Before she could answer and, amazed at how quickly the bush telegraph had worked, Steve cut across her thoughts.

"Once you're done just leave the paperwork on the flight ops in-tray and you're both rostered off tomorrow and Saturday. I will let you know about standby for Sunday so go get some rest, you've both earned it.

"Roger that" said Brad as he tidied up the flight deck and put all his charts and approach plates back in his flight bag.

Bev replenished the medikit and took the tools and equipment back to the ready room for cleaning before storing. Checking off the medications chart and the pain puffers she had received from the Ambos, she locked them away in the used locker so they could be checked with Alice before being put into service.

After a quick wash and change out of flight overall she sees Brad heading out near the front door.

"See you for the next adventure BEBE" said Brad as he headed for his car smiling to himself. Making her way to her car, she noticed Steve was still up in the tower closing off the day and she felt a pang of guilt for not sticking around to help him file the MIRs (medical information reports) and the Worksafe report from the Abercrombie farm incident.

She was tired and the adrenalin was wearing off as she headed for her home in her old car home. Going over the day, she thinks I must follow up on the Abercrombie stuff.

She was sure that Alfredo would recover, but his injuries were not consistent with the evidence of just a fall. Based on the brief chat she had with Armando she suspected there was more behind this incident than she was aware of.

It would also be interesting to see what analysis revealed about the lumps of timber revealed, especially the on with blood on it.

The conditions at the workers' campsites were another thing that was nagging her as she headed down the almost deserted road passing grain trucks heading to the silos at the rail head in town. Harvest and muster were busy times for the community and very important for the local economy.

Pulling into home her phone rang. It was Steve just letting her know he was filing the reports plus one more to the health department about the Abercrombie farm workers situation that he had constructed with her notes. They briefly discussed the content and she was satisfied with it but offered to come in if needs be before hanging up.

Mrs. Buggles

It had been a good move for Bev when she moved into the flat at the back of Mrs. Buggles old house. Between the town and the airfield, it was an ideal location at the end of a lane up on a hill away from the main road.

Mrs. Buggles, or Mrs. B as most people knew her, was always up on the day's events before Bev could say a word. She must have a radar or something, but her tone was always kind and caring and she often made Bev dinner which she enjoyed with a cold beer from the fridge.

Tonight, after dinner they relaxed on the front verandah watching the moon rise and the grain trucks heading down the road with their lights blazing. It was an almost surreal scene with the dust catching the beams of light and creating patterns as the trucks passed by in the distance.

Thankfully, Irene Buggles' place was well removed from the main road and Bev's granny's flat out the back was a haven for her. Irene knew that once Bev went there, she wanted her privacy, and she respected that. She had a kindly habit of always greeting Bev with a cuddle and her scones were to die for when she made a batch for Bev to take to the team at AeroMed.

Bev was very happy living with Irene as her landlord, but she knew someday she would want her own place. The money from the sale of her mother's place was safely banked and earning a modest rate of interest. She had looked but couldn't find anything that suited her and Oliver Bacon, her pet 2-legged pig that still lived at Sams place.

Irene had never pushed her about leaving but was always looking to match make. It was an endearing and well-known habit she had. In her mind you had to be connected to a man to survive.

Her husband of 40 plus years had passed away some years back with a chronic lung condition that was typical in the district and thought to be associated with the dusty environment. Bev had vowed to investigate that when she first heard the stories about the number of deaths from Irene, but time and work had precluded her from that mission.

Sitting back in her chair, Bev was overcome with a tiredness she had experienced before. She could not explain why she was feeling it now as today had been routine except for the Abercrombie farm thing, but she knew she was close to sleep.

Excusing herself she bade Irene good night and headed for her granny flat out the back. Laying on the bed before showering she reflected on the day and her chat with Amy.

Their backgrounds were similar, both nurses with similar experience. Amy suffered reputational damage when she rebuffed the advances of a clinician who, in an act of revenge, brought a malpractice claim against her. It was thrown out, but the damage had been done and her reputation was put in question.

Amy had done what Bev had by moving to the country as a district nurse. As Amy comically put it, they took anyone who could bandage and smile. Bev felt a kindred spirit in Amy and thought they could be friends. Sleep took over and she awoke with a jolt around midnight still dressed and lying on the bed.

She was sweating and had a slight headache. The bad dreams seemed to be back, and she wondered if her chat with Amy had triggered the old memories.

Stripping off she ran a shower and stood under it for some time. Seeing her reflection in the nearby mirror she questioned herself. What's wrong with me, why can't I find happiness and love like everyone else she whispered to herself while studying her naked body in the mirror.

Tears began to well up in her eyes as she crouched down in the shower stall. She shook with emotion remembering the hurt she had felt at the rejection by her colleague over the events in the city. She could never forgive herself for being so foolish as to believe she was anything more than a plaything, to be cast aside and disgraced. She remembers the wife's words which had come true when she said I will ruin you.

Mary had been the only one to stand by her and help her as her mother's health deteriorated until she finally died leaving another void in Bev's already barren life. If it wasn't for Mary, she would most likely have taken her own life. Mary had visited her in the country on a couple of occasions but the distance and the improving situation with Bev had meant she had not been around for some time. She missed Mary and their talks but felt that maybe Amy could fill that void.

Mary and her husband had planned to come up before Christmas in a month or so and she was looking forward to that more than ever now that the bad thoughts had come back.

It was nearly 1 am when she realised, she was not able to sleep and put on a robe and stepped outside to enjoy the night air and quick cigarettes but the bugs were too much for her so she opted for a cup of tea and a few moments on her computer. There was nothing on her email or messages except the usual adverts for junk, so she scribbled a few notes in her journal about the day's events and the bad dreams and lay down on the bed again.

Her thoughts ran to old boyfriends and sexual adventures she had in her younger days, but the image of the married doctor kept coming back to her ruining the good memories. Sleep finally overtook her around 2.30am and she slept soundly until her phone rang and woke her up.

Good morning, Bev, it's Amy, are up for that coffee and a spot of girlie time.

Still half asleep she answered, sure let me get some brekky and I will meet you at the roundup café.

Brekky? Girlfriend, it is almost lunchtime.

Looking at her nurse's watch on the side table she gasped. Oh, shit I've slept through.

No worries girlfriend, see you at the roundup in say an hour?

Wondering how she managed to oversleep she checks her phone and noted a couple of messages from Steve and one from Amanda Johnson the regional Worksafe manager and another from a Dr Raoul Zambi from the district hospital which worried her. She hoped that everything was ok with Alfredo.

A quick face wash and some makeup she dressed in her favourite jeans and shirt. Straightening herself out in the mirror she noted she still had a good figure but was a little heavy in the butt. Perhaps a little bit of gym time might be in order. Grabbing her handbag and phone she headed out and waved goodbye to Irene as she passed her hanging out some clothes over in the yard.

Yelling after Bev Mrs. B says

"Leave your washing on the verandah and I will run it through the wash today,"

"OK, thanks, I'll put it out now, says Bev, going back into her little flat and bringing out the hamper and remembering to give herself a splash of Channel 5 perfume on the way out.

Mrs. B waves, "You had a good lay in, must it have been a big day pet?

"Sure, was Irene and thanks for doing my washing, I owe you one."

"No, it's no bother pet, you go and enjoy yourself. Big date maybe?" Mr. B says smiling.

"No Irene, I'm having coffee with Amy Forest and doing a little girl shopping."

"Oh, that will be nice, she is a lovely lady, and I hope her son is ok."

Walking to her car, she suddenly stops and turns around.

"Irene, how did you know about Amy son's injury?"

"Oh, he is always hurting himself with those stupid bikes. Must worry his mother to death at times. The word gets around about who's in hospital here and the Forests are well known. Good people they are."

Nodding and smiling at herself she walks to the car and jumps in. Heading down the laneway to the main road she calls the Dr from the hospital who had called her earlier, but he is not available. A quick call to Steve produces the same answer but she manages to get hold of Amanda from Worksafe as she joins the main road into town.

Amanda had some questions for Bev about the Abercrombie farm accident and the injuries noted on the MIR (medical Information Report) that she wanted to discuss and wondered if Bev could drop by her office in town so they could discuss. Apologizing for disturbing her day off she said it was important and she could do it anytime she is free.

Driving on Bev was more than a little curious and a bit concerned. Had she stuffed something up? Was there more to this? Only time would tell and she made a note to herself to be cautious at the meeting. Pulling into the Roundup Café she saw Amy waving to her from an outside table.

CHAPTER 6

———◆◇◆———

Handsome Stranger

The Outing

Amy sat smiling as Bev as she approached.

"Looks like you need a rest girl" she says as Bev sat down.

"Absolutely, I've never overslept like that before."

"I get it. I know you're used to the stress and strains of the work you do, been there myself but sometimes the ups and downs of the day compound themselves in your brain and the body just says enough is enough. Make sure you give yourself some time and rest after those heavy days. I'm sure you're suffering from your run in at Abercrombie place al. says Amy."

"I think you're right but it's not my first rodeo and I'm surprised it has affected me that way. Can I also confide in something with you?"

"Sure, nurse to nurse or friend to friend"? says Amy.

"A bit of both Amy, apart from Steve and Alice, you're the only one who knows the problems I had in the city and the aftermath of that.

"I had those bad dreams again last night and woke up in a sweat around midnight. So that's the friend-to-friend bit. Also, I had a call from Amanda Johnson at Worksafe who wants to talk to me about the Abercrombie farm accident. I've never had that happen before should I be wary?"

"Bev, I know what you're going through and how tough it can be. I hope our chat on Aircraft yesterday didn't trigger anything but if you have those thoughts again, call me day or night, OK. I hope we are going to be good friends and that's what friends do, don't hesitate if the thoughts come back. I know you mentioned Mary, but she is a long way away and I'm here anytime you want to chat.

"Now what was the nurse-to-nurse thing? Oh yes Amanda. She is a friend of mine and an ex-nurse, so I doubt there is any problem for you. She is a good operator, and you will get on fine with her. Probably just wants to clear up a few things but take your body cam footage with you as I'm sure she will want to see that. If you like I can come with you to ease the introductions."

"That would be great", says Bev still a little apprehensive.

Anyway, back to our girlie day, its lunchtime and they do a mean schnitzel here if you're up for a big meal" says Amy.

"Thanks Amy, I will just go with a salad of some sort. I saw myself in the mirror this morning and I'm carry saddle bags around the butt, so I think I need to get back in shape".

"Girlfriend, you look great, wait till you have a couple of kids says Amy patting her thighs". They giggle and order lunch, continuing their discussions and finishing their coffees Amy says.

"you're coming with me. I think we need to do something with your look babe".

Some hours later, after Amy had introduced her to the local hairdresser and beauty parlor where she gets a makeover and then on to the dress shop where both have fun choosing outfits. It's late afternoon when they appear from the shops, laughing and giggling like a pair of students. They decide it's time for an ice coffee at the Roundup café and start heading in that direction.

A passing car honks its horn and waves to the two women. Bev says, "That makeover seemed to work then."

"Oh, that was just my brother-in-Law, Charlie. Probably on his way to check on his engineering business in town. I will give him a call when we sit down and see what he is up to. You should meet him, you two would get on well and he is single." She says winking.

"Oh no you don't Amy, not match making like the town Bugle Mrs. B are we."

"No, never, me no, let's get that iced coffee. Then we can see about your appointment with Amanda. she says with a wry smile on her face.

"Shit, Id almost forgotten about that."

"Let's get that iced coffee. Then we can see about your appointment with Amanda Stop worrying or you will ruin the makeup with that frown. You can call Amanda whilst I chat with Charlie who should be here soon. Says Amy with a wink.

"Hang on miss match maker, when was that arranged" says Bev with an indignant look on her face.

"Oh, I just made a quick call whilst you were being tarted up. Anyway, I need to talk to him about some farm stuff so you can just look the other way even though you might find that a bit hard, he is a bit hunky, or so I'm told."

The plan agreed they happily set off for the Roundup Caffe and sitting down inside Amy orders a couple of large ice coffee Supreme's.

"My treat she says these things are to die for and forget your diet for a while babe."

The laughter flows back and forth as they enjoy each other's company and the sumptuous ice coffee Supreme's.

Bev's call to Amanda sets a time for her to meet at 4.30 pm and Amy announces you're going to meet my hunky brother-in-law, for a chat on his way back to the airport to pick up his R44.

Looking bemused, "what's an R44 Amy?"

"Sorry, that a Robinson helicopter. A 4-seater that he uses on the farm. It's at the airport for a quick service after the muster work it did but shouldn't have as the 22 had a problem".

"Oh, I see, does he fly it" says Bev,

"Yes of course, they are practically the main mode of transport on the big stations, and he has nearly 50,000 acres with cattle and sheep on them. I'm sure you will get an invite out there one day the way you look today, I would say it's certainty Charlie will want you to visit."

Feeling like she had been set up but it may just be what she needs and a change of scenery and company would be great. It was about then a tall handsome man in an Akubra hat walks over to the table. Holding out his hand to Bev, He says, Hi Amy, this must be BEBE, I take it.

Bev is struck by his gently touch and well-spoken words shaking her hand. Looking at Bev he says I see she has been leading you astray with those Ice Coffee things she loves. I'm sure Tom will forgive her but it's just between you and me Amy he says winking.

His presence overwhelmed her and Amy could see the sparks starting to fly between them as he sat down.

"I like your new name nick name Nurse Anderson. BEBE suits you" he says smiling at her a little longer than would be polite.

"So, Bev, how come I've not met you before" he says flashing his blue eyes and ordering a flat white coffee.

Recovering her composure Bev responds "Well, I guess we've never had a need to visit your farm or someone else has done it."

Folding his hands but fixing his gaze at her he replies

"I think you're right Bev, its generally Alice Rogers who was out to our place when we've had the odd accident but I think I might request you in future. Who's your pilot?"

"Brad Evans" she says looking deep into his eyes,

"He is a great pilot and a friend of mine from back when I was learning to fly. I still have a beer with him from time to time but say hello when next you see him."

"I certainly will," said Bev. The eye contact stays but the pause in conversation is broken by Amy.

"Hey Charlie, I'm still here you know. I've got an idea. Sean is coming out of hospital tomorrow and I was thinking how would it be if you took us back to your place for the weekend. Maybe Bev could come too if that's ok."

Charlie sat for a moment and said,

"it's Friday tomorrow and that could work but let me see how Andy is getting on with the Robinson before I commit. I could use a hand with the girls who are on school holidays as you know and getting a bit restless.

"Bev, I would love to have you come as well but I will need to check the weight and balance after all the iced coffees you two have been having". as Amy hits him in the arm.

"Just ignore him, he is very rude like his brother. We better make tracks Bev if we are to get to that meeting" says Amy standing up as Bev reaches for her purse.

"The iced coffees are on me Bev" says Charlie gently holding her arm. "I will let you know later about tomorrow."

"Can I give you my number, Charlie" says Bev looking up into his deep blue eyes and handsome face.

"No need to BEBE, I've already got it, thanks to Amy" who was standing in the background smiling like a cheshire cat.

"That name seems to have stuck," he says, gradually letting go of her arm and heading to the counter as Bev stood with her mouth open unable to speak watching him walk away.

"Come on Bev, put your tongue away and let's get to that meeting", We will go in my car as by the looks of it yours is on its last legs". say Amy grabbing her arm.

Thinking to herself as she jumps into the sumptuous seats of the land rover, I must do something about that soon. So, tell me Amy, how come you have this car in town?

"Long story Bev, we keep this one at the airport hangar so we can come and do our shopping. It's not the latest model but it does the job, and we also lend it out to visitors and others who come to see us at the farm. Charlie often uses it when he is in town but prefers his old ute to get around in. He is not into badges and flashy cars, and you will find he is very uncomplicated."

"I look forward to having the opportunity to find out more Amy," says Bev grinning ear to ear and causing Amy to giggle in the knowledge that she was impressed by the handsome Charlie.

"You go girl, he needs experiences of the kind I think you're talking about Bev," smiling naughtily across the cab at Bev.

"You are naughty Amy"; they laugh aloud as they head into the Worksafe office carpark.

Worksafe

As they enter the office there is a call out from the mezzanine attracting Amys attention.

"Amy, up here". A short plump lady waved for them to come up stairs.

"Long time no see Amy, I guess your Bev". I'm Amanda Johnson, so has this one been leading you astray today Bev". she says holding out her hand and smiling.

"Most definitely Amanda good to meet you" says Bev feeling more relaxed as they are ushered into Amandas office.

"Okay, thanks for coming, Bev, I know it's your day off but I have a few questions about your time at Abercrombie farm and your patient Alfredo. I don't suppose you have the body cam video from the day?"

"I can call it up off the cloud for you if needs be" said Bev working some magic with her phone. I will send you a link.

Sometime later after having watched the video and several questions later it's clear that Worksafe has a case to put and wants to do further investigations.

"This is going to be a tricky one, as the Abercrombie's have some weight in this town and I want to be sure before we go ahead further. The hospital has also reported unusual injuries to his leg and face that are not consistent with the accident as per your report and the position the patient was in when you reached him. He has severe chest and stomach, bruising a damaged eye socket and bruising around his legs all of which look consistent with a beating."

I got the timber you bagged up at the farm and it's gone off to the police regional lab who we've notified of our suspicions but in case you don't know the sergeant is close to Jack Abercrombie and has most likely told him of my report and your MIR report."

So, that means, it's likely he will fight back with something against AeroMed and Bev if he is true to form. However, is it ok if I share your footage with the health guys as I think there are some issues with the workers camp they will need to look at. I've also had a call from Clive sanders the aviation authority local manager who wants to see any footage you have and wants to talk with your pilot."

Bev by this stage is getting a bit concerned. Could it all be happening again? Amy senses her discomfort and puts her hand on her arm.

Seeing that Amanda responds "it's Okay Bev you're not in any trouble and I think we may be able to nail those cowboys who have been getting away with murder out there for years.

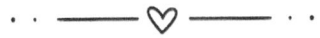

Reassurance

After the meeting was over the ladies walked back to the car but Bev is not comfortable, and Amy reassures her that all is well, and they discuss the possibilities with each other as they head back into town to pick up Bev's car. On the way they drop by Charlie Forests engineering shop to find him busy working on a large pump with his guys.

Looking up he says, Ah two beautiful ladies to grace my humble workshop. Turning to the guys, he instructs them to tidy up the work and head off for the day. Nods tell him they are all in favour of it and ask if he is coming for a beer when he is finished.

"Thanks, but not tonight guys, I've got to fly tomorrow,"

Turning to the ladies he announces that the Robinson will be ready later today but he would rather stay in town and fly out with the ladies and Sean in the morning if he is released from Hospital.

"I was wondering if you two ladies would like to have dinner with me tonight at the roundhouse."

Amy is quick to jump in, "sorry Charlie, I've got to visit Sean and hopefully check him out of the hospital and get him back to the motel as well as arrange his meds, but you two should have dinner", smiling and quietly winking at Bev.

"That would be great, Ok pick you up at 7pm Bev."

Still a bit bemused by what just happened, she stutters.

"Okay, but do you know where I live?"

"Of course, Bev, I do my homework, smiling at her with his perfect teeth and deep blue eyes. So, seven o'clock, ok?"

"Ah, sure ah, what should I wear?"

"What you've got on now is just great pretty lady."

Amy hides her secret smile as they walk back to her car.

"That sounds good, have fun tonight if you know what I mean. she says.

Bev punches Amy lightly on the shoulder,

"you're awful and that was another setup wasn't it, Amy."

No, not at all girl friend says Amy giggling. Take it slowly and enjoy yourself Bev.

The trip back to the car was uneventful with both ladies swapping first date stories and giggling as they went. After dropping Bev off at her car with her packages she heads back to the workshop to brief Charlie of the sensitivities surrounding Bev and as always, he is considerate and obliging knowing his sister-in-law has his best interests at heart and those of her new friend Bev.

Alfredos injuries

On the way back home, she gets a return call from the ER doctor who tells her that Alfredo has been asking for her and that his health position is not too good but he should recover.

Bev doesn't hesitate and turns around to head to the hospital where she meets up with Dr Raoul who briefs her on Alfredo's condition as they walk to the ward. It appears he has suffered a blow to the head, lost teeth and had severe bruises on his body and a possible broken leg.

Entering the room Alfredo lights up and greets her with his angel of mercy statement whilst holding out his hand. Dr Roule explains that he is hesitant to speak about his injuries for fear of retribution on the others at the Abercrombie camp. He thinks that Bev might be able to persuade him and says that he can interpret if needs be, or he can get a fluent Spanish speaker in to do it.

Turning away from the bed towards the Dr she says I will need to record it on my phone if that's OK?

The doctor agrees and the discussions begin with the Dr interpreting between the two. It appears that Alfredo had complained about the conditions and the poor state of the housing and food to the supervisor. He had called Brian Abercrombie who came over with one of his henchmen and listened whilst Armando interpreted what Alfredo had to say.

When he had finished Brian hit him and he fell to the floor. Armando had tried to help but was pushed aside as he went to help Alfredo up. It was then that the henchman jammed his hand into the machine and went ahead to kick him until he was unconscious.

Bev stood up turning off the recording.

"Doctor, you know this is a case of assault don't you."

"Yes, I do but when I reported it, I was told to keep it to myself and the police never showed up. As Alfredo was calling for you, I thought it best we follow the process we have just done in case there are further repercussions. I've informed the head of the hospital, who doesn't seem interested, so I'm not sure if this poor fellow will ever get justice."

"Thanks, doctor, for your care and concern, I will see what I can do, and I will come back to visit him in the morning. Meantime I'm sure you will take good care of him."

"Please call me Roule,", yes, we certainly will take care of him and get him back to full health. After that I don't know what's going to happen to him." the doctor says

CHAPTER 7

───◆◇◆───

Could this be it?

First Date

Noticing the time Bev hurried out the door of the hospital. Realising she has just enough time to get home, freshen up and be ready for Charlie to pick her up. There was a sense of excitement as she headed home down the highway but as she turned into the laneway leading to Irenes place the car spluttered and died.

That's just what I need now she thinks. I knew this damn car was on its last legs but why now? Getting out she kicks the car, hurting her foot in the process.

"Bloody car, couldn't you have just waited to die at my doorstep?"

They had no choice but to walk the rest of the way up the dusty lane to Mr. B's. High heels and her new dress would likely be ruined but she still had the old clothes she had worn to town in the back of the car before they went shopping. The small car was not the most proper place to get changed but there was no other choice so she had just managed to wrestle the new dress off as she took a breather before slipping her jeans and shirt on when a knock on the window alarmed her.

A male voice from outside the slightly steamed up windows asked if she was all right. Covering the private bits Bev hesitantly stammered out her reply.

Yes, fine thanks.

Okay, I will see you at the house and then, and the voice and the car disappeared into the evening. Her mind shot from one thing to another as she struggled to get her jeans on and button up her shirt. Bev looked all over the car but couldn't find her sneakers figuring she must have left them at the shoe shop. She was not going to make it up the lane in high heels so she resolved that socks would have to suffice.

The gravel and dust were making her progress slow and painful but she doggedly pushes on until a set of headlights came down the hill toward her and pulled up beside her. It was Charlie in a not so new pickup truck.

"What are you doing Bev?" asked Charlie leaning across the cab of the truck.

"Oh, me, just taking a walk in the evening with my shopping" she said with an air of quiet confidence and normality.

"I see, I waited at the house with Irene thinking you would pull up soon so when you didn't appear I drove back down the lane to see what happened not expecting to see you tip toeing in the dirt with shopping bags. What happened to the car?" said Charlie with a smile on his face?

It all caught up with her and she felt foolish in front of this lovely man she barely knew but hoped to. The tears ran down her face as she sat down in the dirt and put her head on her knees.

"It's all a bloody mess, I can't get anything right and I feel so foolish. The car died and had to change and ..." the tears flowed and she sobbed with her head on her knees and her makeup running.

Charlie was beside her with his arm around her shoulder and his fingers to her lips.

"It's okay, Bev, you're okay and we are going to have a lovely evening together. he said.

Standing up he took her hand and helped her to her feet. The makeup from the beauty parlor had run and was mixed with the fine red dust on her tear-stained face.

"I must be a sight," said Bev trying to recover her composure and wipe away the tears.

Gently guiding her into the passenger seat of the car he passed her some tissues and wet wipes from the glove box. Bev appreciated both items but thought it a little unusual to find such gently things in the glove box of a working vehicle.

"Thank you, Charlie," she murmured looking up into his handsome face close to hers and ripples of emotion and joy running over her.

Back at Irenes shortly thereafter and having gained her composure she turned to Charlie,

"I'm sorry it looks like I've ruined the evening so perhaps I can take a rain check?"

"That your call Maam" says Charlie in a southern drawl accent that made Bev laugh and reply.

"Well thank you kind sir" in a similar accent. As she headed into the gate Charlie stopped her and again in a southern accent he said,

"Not so fast my pretty one, you all got some boots in there."

Bev was stunned but replied, only my work boots.

With a look of authority on his face he put his hands on her shoulders and said.

"Right, go get cleaned up a little, don't change, just put your work boots on and a hat if you've got one and bring a jacket as well, you're not going to stand me up miss, now scoot."

Irene was on her front verandah and smiling ear to ear as Bev passed her heading to her flat.

"Thanks for the lamb and the jam Charlie. Do you want to come in and wait for her?"

"No thanks Irene, I need to tidy up the old ute before she returns."

Irene headed inside thinking of the wonderful gossip she had an exclusive on for tomorrow.

It wasn't long before Bev emerged and had tidied up her tear and dust-stained face and with a broad smile she skipped down the path displaying her work boots from AeroMed and the clean country women's shirt she had bought in the city before coming to the town in the hope that she would fit in.

However, she found that most ladies wore hi visibility work wear and she stood out instead of blending in. She had tied her hair back and had an AeroMed baseball cap with her ponytail out the back.

Turning in front of Charlie she says "Well?? Is this, OK?? I'm guessing we are heading for some fast-food joint, right?"

Taking her all in Charlie whistles. "You look like wonderful pretty lady. Fast food, no but casual food, yes. Trust me, you're going to have a great time. you're certainly going to shine", he said as he opened the ute door for her and handed her a bunch of flowers he had hidden behind his back.

Yellow rose, what was it they said about yellow flowers thought Bev.

Sliding into the driver's seat he turned to her and said.

"I thought you might like some flowers to brighten your day, which I believe has had its ups and downs. They say yellow flowers are used to spread happiness and joy and it is also the ideal color for symbolizing friendship. I hope these do that and increase your positive energy. You're going to need some energy tonight girl".

Bev sat stunned as the car took off down the laneway. How is it possible that she had met such a kind and sensitive man with such good looks and build and is still single. Maybe my luck is changing? As her mind returned to the moment she said.

"Can I ask where we are going?"

"You can ask but it's a surprise and I hope you like to dance."

"Dance!! In these clothes and boots?" says Bev staring at Charlie who was smiling from ear to ear

"Trust me, city girl, you're perfectly dressed for dancing where we are going. Hope you like steak and beer?"

"Sounds intriguing, can I at least ask where we are going?"

"It's a place called the Ranch and to get you in the mood and give you a clue here some music" he says flicking the radio on to a country and western station and tapping the steering wheel as they headed out of town.

Bev's curiosity was put aside as the thought of spending the evening with this wonderful man overtook her curiosity and she didn't really care where they were going as she continued to glance sideways at Charlie.

It was dark when they pulled into a car park outside a country-style restaurant with music coming from inside. The smell of BBQ meat met her nostrils as they headed into the place. There was a dance floor with couples cruising around the floor in graceful swings and circles. The bar had booths and bar seating was full as Charlie guided her to a booth acknowledging the locals who waved hello as they passed.

Sitting down a girl in a cowgirl outfit came over with a tray and asked what they would like to drink. Looking at Bev he said,

"Can I order for you?"

Nodding agreement as she had no idea what they served but it looked like beer was the main tipple and steak the main food. Charlie ordered them.

"Maryanne lets have 2 porter house steak specials and a mule kicker beer for Bev and Coke with ice for me."

"Not drinking tonight Charlie" says the server.

"No, I'm flying in the morning."

Nodding the server headed off to the kitchen. Charlie explained the meal and the beer and the stares they were getting from the patrons. They've not seen me in here with a lady since my wife died and of course everyone knows BEBE the flying nurse but they've never seen her out of character and casual like tonight.

Night moves

The evening progressed and they swapped stories and got to know each other over the noise. The beer was a wonderful offset to the enormous steak and buffalo wings that Bev struggled through. They were relaxing with a coffee when the lights on the dance floor went up and the MC announced its boot scooting time folks and Charlie grabbed a reluctant Bev to head toward the dance floor.

"Come on, you will love this, just follow me, it's simple."

The music kicked off and the lines of folk began to move. Charlie held her hand and helped her through the steps as the music took over and Bev got in the swing of the simple repetitive steps. Walking off the floor clapping she turned to Charlie and grabbed his arm.

"That was fun, thanks."

"Told you you'd have fun and were dressed appropriately." Said Bev hanging close to Charlies strong arm as they headed back to their booth.

As they walked back one of the band members stopped Charlie and asked if he would sing tonight.

Not tonight, Fred, sorry. Bev grabbed his arm,

"Hey, you took me out of my comfort zone so it's your turn, get up there she says.

"Come on, says Fred, let's get it on" as he drags Charlie off to the stage.

Bev was curious about this other side of the man she was becoming increasingly attracted to. The music started and Charlie strummed his guitar and sang a Kenny Rogers song with more than average talent. The audience sang the chorus and he certainly had a stage presence. Finishing the song the audience applauded and Charlie waved as he left the stage.

"So, when were you going to tell me you're a country and western star Charlie" say Bev.

"I'm just an amateur who messes with music. You might get to hear me sing a duet with my daughter when you come up to the station." Says Charlie smiling and slightly embarrassed.

"I certainly look forward to that she says.

The rest of the evening was a mix of chat and banter and culminated with a swing dances set that Bev enjoyed and finished with a long slow dance together. Having his arms around her and the closeness during the slow dance had her thinking of more intimate things she would like to do with this wonderful man.

The evening was ending and the band played its last song as Charlie whirled her around the floor and bent her back in a final flurry of activity The smile on his face dazzled Bev as he looked down into her eyes and held her there for a longer time than was normal with that dance move.

You can let me up now, says Bev with a glint in her eye and a feeling she would like a hug to finish off the evening of dancing, but it wasn't forthcoming as he stood her up and his face changed.

Sorry, I was a bit distracted. The look on his face told Bev that she was the ghost of his dead wife at that moment and that he still had not let her go. Making his apologies he headed to the band telling her he was going to arrange to have her car picked up in the morning by one of the guys who has a car trailer and have it dropped off at his workshop to see if it's fixable. Looking slightly embarrassed, he headed off leaving Bev to head back to the booth and tidy herself up.

Deep in thought Bev was visiting her own ghosts. The city affair had ruined her life and her reputation, and she wondered if that had tainted her potential for a relationship with Charlie. Perhaps he might think of her as easy or loose or an insane type that latches onto any available, vulnerable male. She remembered Amys advice about taking it slowly and she could see why she had said that. Clearly Charlie was still not over his dead wife.

NIGEL

Her thoughts were interrupted by a drunken voice close to her as a male figure slid into the booth beside her, a voice shook her out of her thoughts and sent a shiver down her as she realised it was the barefoot pilot she had seen the day before at the regional airport,

Well look who we have here Al, he says moving closer to Bev as she moves further around the semicircular booth to escape his attention.

"Little miss flying nursey no less" he says. "I think I need some treatment, how's about taking some semen samples babe" he says with a giggle whilst his friend standing outside the booth smirks. She moved right around the booth to the other side with Nigel following her and his friend blocking her exit.

"Don't be like that nursey, where's your bedside manner. Al and I can show you an injection you will love, trust me" he says grabbing her left forearm. "I think you owe me a little loving sweetheart. Even though I'm not a big city doctor like your last fling, I can show you a good time" he says as he bends to kiss her neck.

Bev's brain is screaming in disgust and revulsion at the drunken obnoxious little man and his friend blocking her way. The fight or flight adrenaline was flowing. Suddenly she recalls the self-defense training they had all had following the tragic rape and death of a nurse on a remote clinic. It had changed everything about these clinics and Bev had taken the lessons seriously. Remembering the moves, she sprang into action.

Bringing her right hand down sharply on Nigel's elbow and elbowing him in the face with the now free left arm, Nigel reeled back in the booth. His friend, Al, had moved in to block her move and tried to grab her shoulders and hold her down till Nigel recovered. A sharp upward palm strike to his chin sawing him reel back and gaining her feet she swept his legs out from under him with a swift move that saw him fall and hit his head on the adjacent table.

She felt Nigel's stinking breath behind her and his hands on her shoulders.

"Okay bitch, you want to have it rough, so let's have it rough then."

Bev's training was kicking in now as she swiftly struck him with her elbow causing him to bend forward and allowing her to break his grip on her shoulders. Spinning around she swiftly put a strong knee blow to his groin and swept his legs from under him as he bent over in pain clutching his groin he went down.

Lying on the ground Bev put her boot on his throat and said.

"If you ever try that again I will break you in half."

She wasn't sure where that tough talk came from but it seemed to cower Nigel who held up his hands in surrender. His friend had blood coming from his head as he tried to get up.

A boot firmly to his groin sent him back to the floor, doubled over in agony.

Stay down if you want to father kids some day she said.

Seeing the commotion Charlie and the bartender rushed over and were standing back in disbelief.

"Are you ok Bev" he says with a tone of concern in his voice.

"Sure, Charlie but I think these two need some first aid."

A couple of the band members had also come over with Charlie and the bartender who was offering Bev a first aid kit. Patching up Als head she noticed that Nigel, still on the ground was bleeding from the mouth slightly and had pissed his pants. Despite objections from him, Bev managed to look at his mouth and noticed he had a front tooth missing.

"You're going to need a dentist; you've lost a tooth. Perhaps some clean underwear also would be good."

Sputtering through the spit and drunkenness he mutters.

"You've not heard the last of this bitch. Do you know who I am?"

I know who you are for sure. You're a pathetic little man who can't hold his drink and pissed his pants after being beaten up by a woman. Try anything like that again and I make you a soprano right. That goes for any of the ladies here or at AeroMed as well. Got it bucko" says Bev staring down at him.

Standing up she has a parting comment.

"Maybe you two would be better off with a blow-up doll than a real woman that your clearly not capable of dealing with. Suggest you go home and have mummy make you some hot milk and cookies and you can jerk off together before going to bed."

She surprised herself saying that in front of Charlie and the others as it was not her way to be crude in public but the words just fell out of her mouth. Surprisingly, the few remaining people who had seen the scene all cheered and clapped as she and Charlie walked to the door. Cheers and Go Girl, high fives and other blown kisses seemed to confirm she had done the right thing.

Walking back to the car, Charlie had been silent. As he opened the door for her, he said.

"Remind me not to upset you. I'm sure your shook you up so you should get some rest and put it behind you."

His gentle touch on her should was comforting and calmed her still adrenaline-fueled instincts.

"I'm fine now Charlie, I recognised one of those creeps as the pilot we saw barefoot at the regional airport. I think his name is Nigel."

Charlie looks at her with affection as he sits across from her in the driver's seat.

"That was Nigel Abercrombie, he is the grandson of Jack Abercrombie and his father Brian runs the Abercrombie spread. He wields some power here but don't worry, you have a lot of witnesses that will stand by you. Also, I think you've just added to your reputation in a very positive way", he says smiling.

"Thanks Charlie Who was the other creep? she says with a soft look in her eyes.

"That's Alan Simpson. That little ferret runs the ABER Motors dealership in town owned by the Abercrombie's. He is a piece of work and known for shaky dealing and parts swapping so I suggest you stay away from that creep.

"He is also connected in some way with the local police sergeant and we suspect there are ongoing corruption issues but nothing has ever been proved. Anyway, put it behind you and have a good sleep. Tomorrow you're coming to the station with us in the helicopter and your car will get picked up early if you leave the keys on the front porch."

They headed off into the night as Charlie explained that she could use the ute whilst her car has been looked at and not to bring too many clothes for the weekend at the Station.

Arriving at Mrs. B's Bev felt this would be the moment for that first kiss but as she subtly leant toward him, he reached out and shook her hand and said,

"I hope you had a good night. I will see you at the base in the morning after the tow guy drops you off now go and get some rest." Waving as he jumped back into the ute and drove away.

Bev stood at the gate for some time as the ute disappeared down the laneway. She was confused and hurt a little. Had she ruined the future opportunities with this man by her violence and crude talk. Was it just to be a friendship or was it as Amy had recommended taking it slowly?

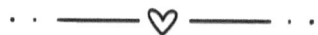

Dissaponting first date

Either way she was disappointed and a little horny after the events of the evening. Her musings were distracted by Mrs. B's asking her how the date was.

"It was great, Mrs. B said Bev as she explained the dancing and the fight over a kind cup of tea and got Mrs. B's thoughts on the Abercrombie's and the corruption in town. It was good to have someone like Mrs. B to chat to but her disappointment at not finishing the night with a first kiss stuck in her mind. She realised she was very tired as she made her way to her garden flat and was quickly undressed and in bed and fast asleep.

A New Day

The early morning sun was gently on Bev's face as she sat on her small porch enjoying her coffee and first cigarette for the day. The gentle scent of Mrs. B's magnolia plants wafted across the garden on a gently breeze. It looks like being a nice day, she thought. The night had not been a comfortable one for her and sleep had been fitful after Charlie's departure.

The morning air seemed to have cleared her head and she was looking forward to her day at the Forest Station with the new man in her life, Charlie. She was still not clear on his intentions but would settle for a friend if that was all there was to be. As the time ticked by, she was thinking she had better get herself ready as the tow truck guys could be here anytime now.

Already showered and with a proper but not overdone amount of makeup she packed a few things into an overnight bag remembering Charlies comments about the weight and balance issues with his little helicopter. Dressed and anxious to get moving she headed for the front gate to await the tow truck guys meeting Mrs. B on the way to the gate.

"Good morning, dear, I hope you slept well and it looks like you're going to have a great day weather wise. "Says Mrs. B

"Yes, it does Mrs. B, I'm hoping to have a good weekend up on the farm and meeting Charlie's daughters".

"I hope it all works out for you dear; Charlie Forest is good man and has suffered a lot in recent years. Take your time with him, he is still suffering from the loss of his wife and I think your still a bit damaged from your time in the city." says Mrs. B,

Bev wasn't aware that Mrs. B knew anything about her problem with an older doctor in the city, but before she could ask Mrs. B with a knowing look put her arm around her and says,

"Its OK dear, Alice told me the story on penalty of secrecy and we conspired to squash any rumour thanks to some misinformation I was able to spread."

Bev was slightly shocked over this revelation but was also grateful that Mrs. B 's rumour mill was being put to a good purpose despite the persistent nagging fear she had that everybody knew of her city affair and problems it had brought.

The comment that that creep Nigel had made last night meant that the knowledge might be further than she thought and perhaps Charlie had heard a twisted version of the story which us why he brushed her off last night. She vowed to tell Charlie the full story when the time was right to ensure he had the truth about her past.

Her fear was not so much about the events but that locals would think they were second best and an escape from problems that she couldn't face. Of course, nothing was further from the truth but in part she had escaped the city and all that went with it as after her mother's death there was nothing left for her there. This place had given her a fresh start and a new career that she loved and she wanted that to be the story.

Reflecting on Mrs.'s comments and the motherly look in her eyes she gave her a hug and said.

"Thank you for that. I love it here so much and just want to fit in."

"You have fitted in dear; your part of the place now so doesn't forget that. Go and enjoy your weekend with that lovely man and remember the old saying. The best way to get over a man is to get under a new one. said Mrs. B winking.

Bev's eyes widened and her mouth opened. She said, "Pardon Mrs. B". she said smiling broadly.

"Oh, I see, you think I've not had my flings and all I do is sit here and fiddle with my garden."

"No of course not, you just took me by surprise" says Bev not meaning anything by her comment.

"It's ok dear, just take your time Charlie OK, says Mrs. B as she looks deeply into Bev's face. Bev could not but have a tear in her eye and gave her a big hug. She was really becoming a mum to her.

"Here is your tow truck dear" says Mrs. B as the large crew cab pickup pulls up with Bev's car on a trailer behind it. The older man driving leans out the driver's window.

"Here you go BEBE, you left it open so we just winched it onto the trailer, handing her a plastic bag with some stuff from inside the car. Ready to go," he asks,

"Off you go, says Mrs. B, I'll look after your stuff and put it aside until you get back. You are coming for tea and scones later Ernie" says Mrs. B winking at Bev as she heads for the back seat of the crew cab.

Bev smiled and winked back with that knowing look that women have when they read each other's intentions.

"Wouldn't miss it for the world sweetheart. I've got some of Forests latest plum jam for you as well."

The touching of each other's hand showed Bev that these two had something going and she was so pleased that Mrs. B had some pleasure in her life with this kindly older man.

"Right then BEBE, let's get you to the AeroMed Base, "Said Ernie as they set off down the laneway toward the main road.

Along the way to the Base Ernie introduced his son bill who was in the band and told her not to worry they will figure out what's gone wrong with her car. As they chatted it became clear that Ernie was a widower and had feelings for Mrs. B as they had been old school days sweethearts but married others. Ernie's son worked for Charlie and was full of praise for the family and their involvement in the community.

It wasn't long 'before they pulled into the AeroMed base car park. Thanks to Ernie and Billy she headed toward the entrance. Ernie yelled after her,

"Well done last night girl, that idiot needed his cards punched". Wave thanks, she headed into the main AeroMed building.

CHAPTER 8

Tough Nurse

Slugger Bev

As she entered the AEROMED lobby she marveled at the speed of bush telegraphs as she headed upstairs with a well-done comment from the receptionist waving as she passed. Passing others on the stairs heading up to the Ops center they all gave her a thumbs up and patted her on the back as she passed. Bev was amazed how quickly the incident knowledge had travelled. Passing the staff kitchen and rest area Alice called out to her.

"Hey Slugger, hope your sticking around for Brekky, the guys want to say something to you OK."

Waving as she headed up to the old ex Airforce control tower, waving her acknowledgement she gave Alice a thumbs up.

Steve was standing looking out across the airfield with his big ex-military binoculars.

"Morning Boss what's happening." says Bev,

Handing her the glass Bev could see a large black helicopter over at the other side of the airfield and further up where the Heli flite hangars were she could see Charlie talking with a man in coveralls as they walked around a sleek little helicopter pointing to things. Charlie looked even better in the daylight with his muscular legs and shorts and strong arms as he pulled on things.

"Okay, Miss, that enough of your perving on Charlie, It's the government Sikorsky I was talking about." Says Steve

Feeling a bit embarrassed she handed the glasses back to Steve.

"So, what the deal with the big chopper" she asks.

"I Don't know Bev, but rumour has it they are headed out to the Abercrombie place. I thought you might be able to recognise whose there and what they are loading", says Steve, handing the glasses back to Bev.

Bev could see several figures moving around the chopper and could see the flight crew and Amanda Johnson from her meeting yesterday. They were loading aluminum cases and There was a man and women in dark uniforms she had not seen before.

Steve gave her a running commentary. "The 2 uniforms are federal Police, immigrations and customs officers. Can't say

I know the others but I think I saw Clive Sanders the local Aviation authority manager there before".

Bev helped him out with her input.

"The lady on the left is the Area Worksafe Manager Amanda Johnson and I'm supposing those are her minions she is ordering around. Those are likely field test kits in those aluminum cases."

"That makes sense, looks to me like a raid on Abercrombie's Place. I've seen a flight plan this morning which is heading in that direction with no end point. That's typical of a Feds raid. says Steve,

Turning to Bev, he could see that she was uneasy and guessed it had something to do with her visit to the Abercrombie place and her run in with Nigel Abercrombie last night. Gently turning her toward him with his hands on her shoulders he sits her down in his chair.

"Look Bev, I know you're what thinking right now and I want you to put it right out of your mind, OK? What you did was by the book and right. What the authorities do with the information is up to them but it in no way would or should have any repercussions for you."

Still not convinced, Bev looks up at Steve with just a hint of tears in her eyes.

"I know Steve but these people have power and I've had some experience of how powerful people work and what they can do even if its outside the legal framework."

Putting his arms around her as she stands, he comforts her in a fatherly way.

"Nobody is going to threaten or intimidate you Bev as long as I'm in this seat, don't forget the amount of support you have in the community also would make that impossible." he says,

Feeling slightly better, she smiles at Steve and kisses his cheek.

"Thanks, boss, I'm feeling better about it now., but what do you think will be the likely outcomes" she says, noticing the big chopper lift off and track along the runway with some radio calls coming through Steves radio systems speakers.

Reaching over to turn it down he says,

"Bev, I think the Abercrombie's are in for a rude shock. They have been running rough shod over this community for years and its perhaps time they were pulled up for their actions." Looking over Bev's shoulder he sees Amy coming up the stairs.

"Morning Amy" says Steve acknowledging her appearance at the top of the stairs.

Strolling over Amy assumes a boxing pose as she approaches.

"Morning Steve, morning slugger," she says tapping Bev on the shoulder. The three laugh at the action and it appears the tension has been broken.

"Alice wants to know if you're ready for Breakfast yet". Says Amy.

"Absolutely aren't we Bev," says Steve. Clapping her hands together Amy grabs Steves' arm and turns to Bev,

"Can you hang here for a little while and don't come down till you hear loud music, ok."

"Pardon, what's that got to do with breakfast? says Bev,

Amy looking stern,

"Listen to me slugger, the boss here is in charge, right? So, he wants you to wait, right?" She says nodding at Steve.

"That's correct, Maam, Slugger is to wait till the music starts." Steve says with a slightly bemused look that he says he doesn't know what's going on either.

Putting her hands up Bev says, "okay, Okay I will obey."

As Amy and Steve head down the stairs Bev turns to look back at the airfield and notices Charlie spooling up the little chopper and heading down the runway and across to the AeroMed helipad. It was a pleasure to watch his delicate touch as the helicopter settles gently on the big H of the helipad.

She was really looking forward to her weekend with Charlie and discovering his world.

Her thoughts were interrupted by the sound of loud music coming from the crew room below the stairs. It was the theme music from the movie Rocky. She had the feeling she knew what was coming. Nothing for it but to face the music so to speak.

Getting in the theme of the music she descended the stairs throwing mock punches and turning as she went to the cheers of the assembled AeroMed team, including everyone from the workshop and a lot of folks who were off duty but had come in for the event. Mrs. B and Ernie were also there, which was a surprise. Charlie had just walked in as she reached the foot of the stairs and the music stopped.

The chief engineer and head of maintenance stepped forward, greeting her with a small object covered with a cleaning rag.

On behalf of all of us here at AEROMED we want to present you with the inaugural slugger award. Removing the workshop rag he handed her a piece of Aircraft alloy, crafted into a plaque with 2 miniature boxing gloves on it and a small propellor in the center with her name, BEBE, on a small plate on the bottom.

Cameras flashed and Bev gave her thanks to everyone with the hint of a tear in her eyes. The cheers and back slaps fell away as Steve pointed out that Breakfast is served with Alice putting some big trays of rolls with Bacon and eggs on them and a comment, come on, don't be shy, it's all got to go so bog in.

Charlie made his way over to Bev and handed her a roll and kept one himself.

"You need to eat before we fly Bev. Did you sleep well?"

They chatted for some time with Charlie explaining his plans for the weekend when Amy strolled over.

"Charlie, Sean, and I won't be coming. Sean wants to work on his bike, and Tom has flown the 172 up ready to take us home. We'll reschedule and maybe meet at the lake for the bird's return. Is that little dirt strip out there still serviceable Charlie," she asks.

"Sure, is Amy, just cleaned it up before muster but I will check it out and give you a call. Bev, where's your baggage, I will meet you at the chopper when you're ready."

Grabbing Amy by the arm as she turned to leave,

"Is this another setup," Bev says smiling.

Walking away Amy says,

"Maybe, Maybe," looking back provocatively and flicking her hair as she went.

"Have a great weekend girlfriend and take it slowly."

Bev, silently mouthing the words, thank you and smiling, she picks up her shoulder bag and heads for the helipad.

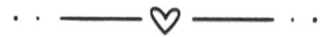

Helicopter experience

The morning was perfect for the flight to the station with clear skies and just a light breeze rustling the trees in the nearby car park. Steve was engaged in conversation with Charlie as he did his preflight of the helicopter so she thought best to leave them to it and just hopped in the right-hand seat to make herself at home in this new experience of flight she was about to hopefully enjoy.

Passing by her door Steve popped his head in and said.

"I won't need you back here till around lunch time Monday. You're going with Dr Web to a clinic at Tagalong station to provide medical support. You're in the wrong seat. Have a great weekend BEBE." Smiling he headed back to the office and the ops room where he mostly hung out.

Bev was puzzled by his comment about the wrong seat but didn't have time to ask why. Maybe she was supposed to be in the back seats. She had always flown in the right-hand seat with Brad so maybe it was a bit presumptuous of her to assume this was the same deal.

Charlie put his head on the door and said with a smile.

"Oh, so you're flying to us today, Maam?"

Looking puzzled Charlie explained that it's the opposite way around with helicopters. Pilot in command in right seat, co in the left. Unless you want to sit in the back but it's full of stuff for the station he explained,

As she moved across to the other seat and he helped her with her seat belt and handed her a headset from a hook behind her.

"I would rather have you beside me" he says his face close to hers as he adjusted her headset and looked deep into her eyes sending shivers up Bev's spine as he touched her arm gently before moving round to the pilot seat.

Charlie made sure she was comfortable and explained the door latches and seat belt operation and briefed her on the flight, asking if she would like him to run through the startup procedure with her giving a checklist. Bev was fascinated with the process of starting the helicopter and getting the rotor speed and other settings to the right point on the gauges as she read out each line on the card.

It wasn't long before the little helicopter was airborne and as Charlie explained they would hover taxi out and leave on the operational runway. As it's just good practice and lets others who might be in the pattern know where you're and your intentions. Bev was amazed at the agility of the little craft and its ability to climb.

Ascending to 2500 feet Charlie completed all the radio work and set up a course for Forest station. She had previously asked him if that was a play on words like afforestation and he had agreed that it was not a mistake. A point which he made again as they headed along the main northern highway. Bev was enjoying this relatively low flight and the wonderful vision she had of the road and the cars and trucks travelling along it.

Charlie explained his reason for following the road was to give her some perspective on their way into his property if she ever had cause to drive it.

The journey continued and Bev was feeling more relaxed and enjoying the journey and a view of the landscape she had not previously been able to see from her seat in the fixed wing Aircraft that only flew this low when approaching land.

The hunk flying her was a definite bonus and she harbored thoughts of where this could lead to.

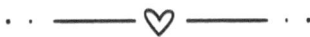

The Local Town

They approached a small town and Bev could see the usual shops and a pub as Charlie pointed them out as his local town. It was sparse but seemed to be a friendly place with some sports fields and parks. As they flew over, he noticed a couple of locals outside a pub wave at them and he waggled the helicopter in response.

Bev looked across at him with a shocked look on her face not having seen the folks on the ground.

"Are we ok" she said holding onto her seat belt.

Sorry, I forgot to tell you, I just acknowledging some friends on the ground, not long to go now, it's just up the road from here." says Charlie,

Minutes later, Charlie brought the little chopper to the hover and pointed out a large signpost which read Forest Station turning here. With a simple movement he headed the chopper off along a winding dirt road explaining it as one of his ongoing projects and how he had spent a lot of time and money on drainage for what was a minor flood plain.

Passing over a gated sign which read "welcome to Forest Station he headed off to the left away from the path to the homestead she could see in the distance.

"I want to show you the station Bev so you will have a better idea of the place and how its runs," says Charlie.

A good sign thinks Bev, as they travel along the boundary fences at low level Charlie pulls up and hovers near various objects and buildings explaining his intricate water reticulation supply system he engineered and the various muster points accommodation.

Waving to the remaining crew finishing the annual muster and packing up, they sped off towards a large body of water.

"That's Lake Edward you can see in the distance. It was named after our great grandfather Edwin Edwards. It has an Aboriginal name as well but the locals still refer to it as Lake Edward. That little hut down there is our boat house and this weekend is the celebration of the return of the birds and we are all going out there for it. I hope you come with us as it's quite a celebration and has some spiritual meaning to the Aboriginal people.

Turning east Charlie announces its time to head to the homestead and meet his girls.

CHAPTER 9

———◦———

Charlies Girls

Meeting the Family

"Bev, we will be landing at the Homestead soon and you will get to meet my daughters. The eldest is Jennifer and the younger one Annabelle. They were named after their maternal grandmother's middle names but please just call them Jenny and Annie when you meet them. I'm sure you will understand they are teenagers and trying to fit in with their peers and it's been hard for them at boarding school over the years since their mother died.

"Jenny is in her final year at high school and wants to become a vet, she spends part of her holiday with Sam at his animal rescue center and the rest of her time in town with her boyfriend Billy, Ernie's son."

"I've met him, nice young man. says Bev, Charlie agrees with a nod.

Continuing his talk.

"Annie has a few more years to go and seems interested in horticulture and often spends time with my brother on his spread, Forest Farm, where they are growing things other than cattle and sheep which is our crop.

"I would like her to come home and attend the local Ag College rather than stay at school without her big sister to help her but she is head strong like her mother.

"I think you're going to like them both. Jenny is more reserved and quieter and she is always studying something whilst Annie is more boisterous and outgoing. She also speaks her mind as you will see so don't be put off by her abruptness. She is also a great cook so expect something good to eat whilst you're here."

First Glimpses of the Homestead

The homestead came into sight as they turned south. It was a beautiful L shaped country style building with large sheds up a short road. The house was surrounded by gardens and lush semi tropical plants that amazed Bev for this dry part of the country. As they came nearer Bev could see a lovely swimming pool with 2 figures lounging in it.

Noticing it Charlie said

"That will be the girls Bev, they love lounging in the pool after they've done their chores. I won't go too close as they hate the downwash when I do. Pulling up into a hover Charlie cancels the SAR watch and settles the chopper down gently on a concrete pad outside of a large hangar.

Turning to Bev as he shuts the chopper down and asks her to hang tight till the girls arrive to take her up to the homestead.

"I've got some stuff to unload from the back seat, so sit tight and wait for the girls to come pick you up.

"No, I'm quite capable chief. I'll help you with it if you just direct me where you want it" she says with a smile on her face.

"Okay, if you want, take the boxes on your side at the back and stack them near the hangar door. They're all going up to the homestead, I will put the Aircraft and other heavy bits away in the hangar and come up and join you later.

Bev was busy stacking the boxes and parcels Charlie had told her were going up to the house when a ute and a kind of golf cart with an alligator painted on its nose.

A tall willowy girl with long fair hair stepped out of the ute. She was wearing a pair of cut jeans; a work shirt tied at the waist with a bikini top underneath. Her outfit was set off by a pair of work boots and an Akubra hat stylishly turned up at the sides. She Was a beautiful young lady thought Bev and this must be Jenny as she strode confidently towards Bev with her hand outstretched as she came closer.

Hi, she said, I'm Jen, you must be Bev, Welcome to Forest station.

Close behind her came a slightly shorter girl in a one-piece bathing suit with shorts over it and like her sister wearing work boots. No less attractive but with shorter hair she shook Bev's hand and said. Hi, I'm Annie and what she said. Charlie had finished moving stuff and walked over. I see you've met the girls Bev says Charlie giving them both a cuddle from behind.

Annie, can you take Bev and these boxes and stuff back to the house and show her to her room so she can freshen up, then start putting the stuff away, it's all marked and there is something in there for both of you but I want to open when we are together OK! Jen, can you help me put the bird away as usual and then we can head back for some lunch after we drop off these pump spares at the number 2 bore on the way back.

Charlie seemed to have mastery of the situation and so Bev nodded and followed Annie to the little 4 seat alligator. Been in one of these before Bev says Annie. Yes, a couple of times on other farms. Do you like driving it? Sure, do says Annie, it's all I've got apart from the farm bikes and Dad is not too keen on my riding them after Sean my cousin and I had an Accident out at the lake. An accident! Says Bev, were you hurt? No, just scratches and bruises but the bikes didn't do too well after they went into the lake and there was a big clean-up job.

In no time they were pulling up outside of the house with its beautiful gardens. Annie explains, they're all remote watered and fertilized thanks to Dad's systems which I'm sure he will bang on about and show you, his map. Looking at Bev with hooded eyes Annie says, try to be interested but when it gets boring suggests he shows you the pumphouse over there which is where the magic happens.

They move into the foyer through an ornate door and Bev notices the detail and craftsman ship with high ceilings and timber floors. Annie is quick to point out that her dad built it with her Mum. Sadness shows in her eyes as she explains some of the intricacies and the solar power and recycled water as they walk down a long passageway.

Opening a door Annie leads Bev into a magnificent bedroom with a large canopy bed. Opening another door Annie shows her the ensuite and the facilities set up for her stay. Bev is blown away with the sheer space and luxury in the remote homestead. Annie, making her apologies, leaves to make lunch whilst Bev sits in the chair looking out toward the beautiful swimming pool and wondering how much better it could get. A quick shower and freshen up the makeup and some fresh clothes and she headed out to find the kitchen and Annie.

Bev was deep in discussion with Annie as she worked her magic with a fresh salad and cold meat lunch platter. Her freshly baked bread smelt wonderful and Bev was amazed at the confidence and skill of this 15-year-old as she swooped around the kitchen making lunch and pouring Bev a cold drink from a large pitcher. This is my special brew Bev says Annie, It's a mix of Mango and Tangerine with a dash of lemon.

We grow some of that here but Auntie Amy and I have a deal with the other bits. She has my recipe and I get unending supplies of her fruit to play with. You can buy the one in town you know but I will give you a carton to take back when you leave.

That's very kind of you to say Bev as the pair chat and appear to bond over recipes and ideas. Bev pitches in to set the table for lunch and is really enjoying this home life atmosphere and Annie's company as the chat and giggle. Charlie and Jenny Walk in shortly after the table is set and Bev and Annie laugh at some inane joke about tomatoes.

Well, says Charlie, it looks like you two have hit it off and it didn't take her long to set you to work Bev. I bet she plied you with her special juice, works every time. You do know she practices witchcraft, he says laughing whilst Annie hits him on the arm.

Over lunch Bev gets to talk more with Jenny and is similarly amazed by her in-depth knowledge of a range of things. She promises to show Bev her lab and darkroom after lunch to which Bev replies she would be delighted. Lunch over, Bev begins to help clear away the plates when Jenny stops her saying, no you're a guest, head out to the verandah near the pool and we will bring out coffee and some of Annies walnut cake.

"Don't argue," says Charlie, taking her arm and leading her out to two comfortable chairs near the pool. "Make yourself comfortable whilst I spread the umbrella." Bev was impressed with the calm and certain way Charlie went about things. It was clear his girls loved and respected him and the affection from both sides showed.

The coffee and walnut cake arrived with Annie asking for feedback on the new recipe for the cake and noting she had made Columbian blend for their coffee which was Dads Favourite.

Departing with a knowing smile that was way beyond her young years she winked at Bev and hurried off to the house leaving the pair alone and discussing how the homestead came into being. Charlie explained that when he first married his wife Jill they had lived with Tom and Amy and Jack Forest Senior and his wife. When Jenny came along it was time to get a place of our own and the family owned this old place as an offset between cropping and cattle.

It was very run down and although it had a small airfield and hangar there wasn't much of a house so I spent weeks out here converting the hangar to a bunk house so we had somewhere to live whilst we renovated the house. Jenny stayed with Jill who went back to work as a district nurse and I worked on getting this place in shape. Fortunately, the family still had a small apartment in town which served as a halfway point for us to meet up and raise Jen. However, it was there that we had Annabel aka Annie and that made things difficult. Over the next 6 months I had my brother Tom and dad help me sort the farm out to a usable standard and Sam, the vet, was very helpful in sorting out the animals and the breeding routines.

Without Sam we wouldn't be talking today as the cattle I inherited were a mixed bag but in very poor condition. Anyway,

Jill and the girls moved into the renovated hangar and we were a family again.

"I will get the girls to take you over to see JAC and explain their special rooms later." Says Charlie

"Jac," says Bev??

"Sorry yes, that's the initials over the door and it stands for Jen, Annie and Charlie. However, some of the young ones call it the Jac off room which is a bit unfair and its never said in my presence but I know" he says smiling.

"I've got to go and finish a few things over at JAC where my office is but please sit here and relax, there's towels in your room if you want to swim. The girls will take you over to JAC and show you, their areas." Charlie smiles like the cat that caught the mouse.

"Thanks, which would be nice and yes, a swim will be wonderful. Before you go, if it's not too intrusive can you tell me about Jill and how you met". says Bev.

"Well, it's still a bit raw even after 5 years. I still see her touches everywhere and feel her presence at certain times. I know that sounds funny but if there is life after death, I'm sure she is around. This pool for instance, she dug this out with a mini backhoe on weekend. I would hear her out here on it at midnight digging away. It's a fiberglass pool of course but the sandstone edges were her idea and she hand laid most of them by herself." says Charlie with a faraway look in his eyes.

"Anyway, to answer your question we met at university when I was studying engineering and she was studying medicine.

We had mutual friends but we hated each other. She thought I was a pompous nerd and I thought she was snobby hippy. She came from an orchard over the ranges that her family ran.

"However, when her mother got ill Jill gave up uni in her 4th year and went home to look after her. She didn't say goodbye as we were barely on nodding terms. We lost touch but after her mother died and within 12 months her father suffered a fall and his health went backwards. Jill asked her brother John, who was in the Navy, if he could help in some way as she had no idea about running the orchard.

"John gave up his military career and took over the farm. Jill managed to convert her med school points and completed her nursing degree and paramedic qualifications. She tried to get positions locally to no avail. When John married, she knew it was time to leave and applied for several district nursing jobs. The one she goes was here."

"Okay, but you weren't the best of friends so what happened?" says Bev.

"I broke my fingers doing some fencing at Tom's place and Amy was away in the city at the time so Tom called the district health services which might have sent AeroMed but in this case they had a nurse close by. That was Jill. I remember her first words when she entered the room. Oh! Shit, It's you! Nice to see you to again snotty bitch I thought."

"So not a good start" says Bev?

"No but she patched me up and drove me to the district hospital where they set it and kept me for a day or so. Amy dropped in on her way back from the city with Tom and took me back to the farm. Charlie says with a sly smile on his face.

"Yes... and then what" says Bev??

"Well, there is this spinsters and bachelors ball held every year in town. Amy convinced me to go against my better judgement but there I was sitting on the sidelines and watching the couple's whirl around the hall when suddenly there was Jill with her hand out inviting me to dance.

"I recall looking at her and thinking how beautiful she was for a snobby bitch and I will just have to put up with her or people will think I'm aloof. Well, we danced until it was time for me to sing some stuff with the band and I recall her looking up at me from the dance floor with her mouth open, a little bit like you did at the Ranch thing, and a look of amazement on her face."

"So that was that eh?" Says Bev.

"No, we didn't see each other for some time but her work association Amy meant she began appearing at family functions and the like."

"That sounds like an Amy ploy to me" says Bev.

"Possibly but over time we became friends and found out our opinions of each other were completely wrong. One day we were out on the quad bikes together and Amy had packed a picnic for us. We sat under a tree and had lunch and when I looked into her eyes, I knew this was the girl for me. My heart melted and we had our first kiss under that tree. The rest was history." says Charlie with a faraway look on his face.

"Thanks for telling me all that Charlie, you must have loved each other dearly and its obvious you've felt her loss deeply" says Bev reaching out her hand to touch his arm.

"Yes, we all did, she was my soulmate, partner, lover and friend and we built this place. When she found she had breast cancer she hid it from us until it was obvious something was wrong. The whole family went into deep depression and she passed away within 6 months leaving an enormous void in our lives. It's been 5 years since she passed but I still think of her every day and visit her grave over there often to tell her what's happening and how the girls are going." clearly the tears are close as Charlie's voice wavers and he looks away.

Putting an arm around him Bev tries to comfort him.

"She must have been a special lady Charlie", says Bev looking up at him and seeing the pain in his eyes, she thinks to herself that Amy was correct, and she needs to move slowly as this man is still in mourning.

Turning to go after a long silent pause between them Charlie heads off saying,

"Relax and enjoy yourself BEBE" waving over his shoulder as he leaves the pool gate and heads off.

She now had a better understanding of this wonderful man and his deep pain. At the same time, she could feel a developing bond with him and whilst it's too soon to use the word love it was a very deep feeling she had for him that she hoped would grow between them.

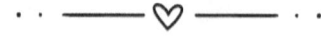

Bonding.

The chance for a swim was an opportunity not to turn down so after Charlie left for his JAC facility, Bev headed for her room to slip into her swimming costume. It had been some time since she had enjoyed the feeling of floating in water as there aren't many swimming holes in this part of the world and the city was not much better.

Standing in front of the mirror in her room she considered her body in the one-piece swimsuit she had brought with her at Charlies prompting. She hoped that Charlie would like what he saw when the occasion presented itself. Moving back and forth she made a mental note to do something about her thighs and butt which seemed to have a life of their own lately. Best wrap that scarf thing around her waist she thought as she left her room.

Heading to the pool and thinking maybe a bikini might have been better but perhaps she would save that for more intimate swims. Her thoughts were interrupted as she passed Jen in the hallway.

Enjoy your swim, and when you're ready Annie and I will take you over to JAC. Smiling back, she agreed that it would be nice and she wouldn't be in long, just a quick dip she explained.

"No rush, just holler when you're ready and no need to dress up," says Jen.

The water was refreshing and cool under the shade of the palms and Bev lay back into the water floating on her back. She had missed swimming as it was one of her favourite outings on better days at the city beach when she was off duty.

She and Mary would head to the beach and the saltwater pool as often as possible. Her mind started to go back to the happier times she had spent in the city. Thoughts of her close friend Mary and her husband came to her mind and she made a note to call her when she got back home to Mrs. B's

Her thoughts were rudely interrupted by a splash which caused her to lose her floating moment and submerge with the surprise of it all. Surfacing, she found herself face to face with a dog in the water with her happily splashing around and another one standing on the pool edge.

Jen's voice came from inside the house,

"Sammy, get out of there you naughty dog."

Sammy was not fazed by the voice or its tone and continued his way to the steps and climbed out shaking himself as Jen appeared.

"I'm sorry he thinks he owns the pool. Come on you two y off to your compound."

"Its OK Jen, he just startled me. Are they your dogs?"

"These two, no way, they're working dogs they've both been on the muster and always very naughty afterwards."

Pointing at the dogs now sitting obediently beside her.

"This naughty boy is Sam and this is his less naughty sister Jess. They are both Kelpies and were born here on the station. Just so you know they're not pets but it's OK to pat them if you like."

Bev had swum over to the edge of the pool and presented a hand to each dog before patting them.

"They seem to like you; they have their own compound just over there; I will get them out of your way so you can enjoy your swim in peace." Said Jen

"No need Jen, I happy to have them around to take a swim with me if they want."

Pushing back Bev calls the dogs into the pool. Without hesitation they both jump in and start happily splashing around with Bev at the center. Jen was smiling broadly and thought that's a plus, she likes dogs as she turned to head back inside.

"Yell out when you've had enough of them" says Jen.

The enjoyable swim was over with the 2 dogs shaking themselves dry as Bev toweled herself off and sat down at the table near the pool. Both dogs seemed to think they had found a friend and came over to sit at her feet. Bev was just ruffling their heads when Annie appeared.

"I see you've met these two rascals", handing Bev some dog treats to give them. This will make you a friend for life she says.

Sitting beside Bev the forthright Annie just came out with it.

"Do you like my dad?"

It took Bev by surprise and the abruptness of the question stalled her response but she had rehearsed an answer which for now escaped her so she just winged it.

"Yes, I do, I think we are going to be good friends and I hope you and Jen will be too."

"If the dogs and Dad approve, I'm sure we will get on fine. Annie says smiling.

"Do you want to sleep with him?" she asked.

This one really threw Bev. She had been warned about Annies's forthrightness and had no answer. Thankfully, Jen arrived at the same time as the question.

"Annie, what a thing to ask. Ignore her she is a little forward, Go and get that tray of stuff and if our guest is ready, we can head over to JAC."

Leaning closer to Bev, the more mature girls whisper to Bev.

"I wouldn't blame you if you do, he is very attractive to older women you know".

Smiling broadly, Bev giggles and says,

"Enough of the old please and yes, he is very attractive but for now we are friends as I hope we are to."

Putting her arm around Bev Jen says,

"I hope we are friends and that this is not your last visit."

Annie arrives carrying a large metal tray with a cover over it. Seeing Bev is curious, Annie explains its BarBQ night. When you've dried off and perhaps dressed come over and we will show you around. Bev had noticed trucks pulling up and a large spit roast being put into action with a pig slowly turning. Thinking to herself this might be a bigger deal than she thought.

Bev headed off to take a quick shower and tidy herself up a little, she thinks, what to wear? So far, it's been jeans and boots or aviation nurse uniform. She had bought a little red dress with a slightly lower than normal neckline. Maybe a bit to Girlie for a BBQ. What she thinks. Slipping into the little red dress she checks herself out in the tall mirror before slipping on a pair of sandals. Well, here goes she thinks as she heads out to find the girls chatting in the kitchen.

Jen is the first to comment, wow Maam, you look hot. Wait till the guys get a look at you out of uniform. Annie, ever forthright says, I think it's for one special guy, winking and grabbing Bev's arm. Come on siren, let's go show you off and look at JAC.

Walking toward JAC the girls explain the veg gardens and Annies's greenhouse. Bev notices the area behind the homestead was filling up with all manner of vehicles, caravans and RVs. Seeing her looking Jen explains the nature of the muster ball and its importance and explains that there is a housekeeper called Esmeralda and her husband Juan who normally look after the cooking and some of the cleaning as well as working with us on this event.

Dad insists we help and do our own rooms as well as our chores. However, she explains that the couple usually head off to town when the holidays come to see their relatives or take a trip. Esmeralda and Juan had been with them since before their mother died, she explains and they love them both like grandparents.

JAC Rooms

TAH DAH says Annie standing with her tray in front of a barn door with a sign above it says just JAC. This is where the fun happens, she says as they enter a large open area, A small stage with a drum kit and some amplifiers sat in one corner. Large pendant lights hung down over the areas with some table and chairs and a lounge at one end. On the other side of the room were 3 large doors with individual letters J,A,C on them.

"Guess which room is whose?" Says Annie.

"I think she can guess Annie says Jen.

"The little door down the end is the toilet and has a little shower as well. That door down there leads to a mud room for boots. On the way in you passed the BBQ pit and pergola. That's where the stuff Annie is holding is bound to the outdoor fridge and kitchen."

THOR WESENLUND

Bev was blown away with the place, thinking it was just an old equipment shed even though Charlie had explained it was their house for some period. A familiar voice from behind her made her turn around to find Charlie admiring her.

"Well now that's what I call a party dress. Have a good swim?" said Charlie admiring Bev's cleavage and figure.

"Yes, thanks and I met Sam and Jess in the pool as well. This place is amazing".

"It's going to get livelier later, perhaps I should have explained beforehand but I guess you can see we are having an end of muster ball and BBQ for the cattlemen and their families if they are with them. Theres plenty of time before the mob arrives so let me show you my office and then the girls can take you to theirs."

"That's a new line sir, but I like it. Says Bev as Charlie guides her toward the door with the Big C on it.

At the door he turns to Bev and says,

"The way you look tonight, Bev, I think you might get more than a few offers." Smiling at her, he goes on to tell the girls to bring the rest of the stuff over for tonight and then show Bev their special rooms.

With a comical salute the girls both head off to the house to get the rest of the stuff for the night's musterers Ball and BBQ. Annie as always has the last say.

"Be good you two"! Laughing as she leaves.

Charlie's office looks more like something from a Star Wars with a big TV screen on one side and a couple of split computer screens on a long desk. In the corner is a cabinet with lots of electronic equipment and flashing lights. The room was on the cool side but not unpleasantly cold. A long window looked out toward the airfield and she noticed a couple of guns on the wall.

"Don't worry, they are just antiques from our grandparent's day and the barrels are lead filled. Of course, we do keep rifles and other weapons etc. but they are all locked away correctly. If you're interested, we might go and do some rabbit hunting with the .22's tomorrow".

"Thanks, but no thanks anyway what's all this stuff" she asks.

Charlie begins a long and detailed explanation of how almost every element of the property can be checked or controlled from here. Pointing to red and green dots on the big TV screen he explains that these are the bore pumps and here you can see the fence checks so I can see any damage and fly out a drone from here to inspect.

The explanation leaves Bev a little dumbfounded and before she can stop herself, she blurts out,

"No wonder the girls thought you are a nerd". Wishing she hadn't said that she began to apologize but Charlie puts a finger on her lips.

"It's OK yes, I am a bit of nerd but what you're looking at is one of the most efficient farms in the country. We sell and export some of this technology to other farmers.

"I think you'll find the apple doesn't fall far from the tree when you see what the girls get up to in their rooms. Looking out the window as he continues his guided tour, he notes that Amy Tom and Sean have arrived as the little Cessna taxis up to the gate.

"They're early he says. I expect a lot more fly-ins this year and of course the Heli muster guys will be here. Anyway, he says pointing back to a large map, here are my water storages and the underground tanks. Also, you will see on Sunday what we did to put water back into Lake Edward and how that has helped the wildlife."

Curious, Bev asks, "So what the big deal with Sunday?"

Charlie points to the big map and Lake Edward.

"It's the return of the bird's event as it's known locally and farther afield. Over the last week or so the birds have come back to make their nests and breed. It's a big event and folks come from all over. We have the little boat shed out there with all the home comforts and the little boat that Jen usually takes over but I think you will get a look chance to use it this year.

"There are Aboriginal ceremonies as well and we always have a campfire and swag party. I'm sure you will love it but it's back to boots and denim unfortunately. The C room tour is over and with Bev suitably impressed Charlie decides to hand her over to the girls for their tour.

Moving out into the main hall to find his daughters he sees Amy and Tom coming through the door. Moving past the stage area Bev trips over a cable and falls. Quickly on his feet,

Charlie catches her and helps her up. Face to face and close to each other the pause is a little longer than normal and the chemistry is flowing.

Their intimate moment interrupted by Amy who says,

"Well, looks like you two are getting along well", winking at Bev who embarrassed begins brushing herself down and blushes.

"Hey Charlie, can you and Tom bring the stuff from the Aircraft over here whilst I chat with Bev."

Knowing this was girl talk time the two men head off to the airfield on their assigned mission. Meanwhile Amy looks Bev up and down.

"Girlfriend, you really have baited the hook, looking hot babe."

Still blushing Bev hesitantly tries to explain the little red dress. Holding up her hand Amy says,

"Stop, this is me remember, I think you have him hooked just don't reel him in too quickly." They both laugh at understanding the meaning in Amy's words.

Jen walks up to the pair and hugs her aunt.

"When you two have finished conspiring we want to show Bev our rooms." Says Jen

Nodding, Amy agrees she must get a lot of stuff ready and how useless Jen's father and Uncle are at organising stuff like this, Amy heads off to find the two men. A parting comment to the pair reinforces Bev's decision to wear a dress.

"I'm going to put my little black dress on so you girls will have some eye candy competition tonight" she says waving over her shoulders as she leaves.

Jen turns to Bev,

"Come on lets go look at my room first."

Entering her special locked room with the big J on the door, Jen explains that no one is allowed in here and Bev will see why as she flicks on the light.

One wall was covered in butterflies and bugs of all types pinned to the wall with tags on them. A long shelf with numerous bottles housing all sorts of preserved snakes, lizards and other things ran down the other wall. Like Charlies room, a large window faces out toward the airfield which Bev later found out was one way glass. One corner had a separate cubicle and beside that was all kinds of camera equipment. A work bench under the window housed a range of scientific equipment including a very impressive microscope.

Jen explained her interest in nature and whether her studies will go toward being a vet or an entomologist. Explaining her photography, Bev is shown an album full of wonderful pictures of local wildlife and birds, Jen explains the importance of the return of the birds and her interest in photography.

Their chat is interrupted by a knock on the door and Charlie asks if he can come in. Permission granted he hands Jen a package. Here you go sweetheart, open it. Unwrapping the long cylindrical package, she jumps to her feet and hugs her dad.

"Thank you, thank you, thank you, Dad."

"I knew you were hanging out for that telephoto lens so I ordered one and it arrived at the workshop whilst I was in town. Call it an early Christmas present but I figured you could get the benefit of it at the Bird thing on Sunday.

Still hugging her dad Charlie winks at Bev, who smiles back with a knowing grin and realising he has a special bond with his girls but the nerdy stuff must have been handed down to the attractive young lady.

"Okay, enough Jen, if you've finished boring Bev, I know Annie wants to take her into her special room. This is quite a privilege you know Bev, not everyone gets to see theses inner sanctums the girls have."

"I feel truly special, and thanks for the privilege, I'm truly blown away." says Bev.

Taking her leave from Jen, who is busy with her new lens Charlie knocks on Annies Door with the big A on it.

"Can we come in its dad and Bev?" The door swings open and Annie in an apron says.

"What's the password?"

Holding out a small parcel he says

"Seeds" and hands Annie the small parcel.

Opening the door wide to let them past Bev sees what can only be described as a laboratory and kitchen combined. There were lots of stainless-steel benches and a couple of microwave cookers as well as a large gas range and big fridge. A large cupboard had racks of things growing and there is a wonderful full smell of freshly baked bread coming from the oven.

"I will leave you two but don't forget to go and get dressed before 6pm. I will need you tonight sweetheart."

"Yes, Dad and ever so thanks for these."

Annie explains that these are south American seeds for a type of plant she wanted to cultivate but it's taken forever to clear them through quarantine so I must be very careful storing and seeding them she says as she puts them into a locked container inside the big cupboard.

Annie then explains that this is her test kitchen and she experiments with different things for Forest Farm and the bakehouse in town. Saying she is just an amateur seems to belie the setup and Bev asked more questions about her interests and plans.

It seems incongruous that such a young girl can be so deeply involved in food science that she remembers Charlie's comment about genetics and the apple not falling far from the tree. Later she was to learn more from Amy about the work Annie has done for and with them on their canned and bottled produce as well as her bakery exploits.

Leaving the room with more than a little insight into the two remarkable young ladies who were obviously working way beyond their years she wondered how she would fit in with that pattern and ambitions. But for now, there was a party to help organise and she headed off to find Amy to see what she could do.

CHAPTER 10

---•◦•---

Life in the bush

The Musterers Ball

B y 6pm the area behind the homestead is packed with vehicles and people. The area at the end of the Airfield was full of Aircrafts and helicopters with some tents rigged under wings and on the helicopter tail booms. Outside the spit roast smelt wonderful as the various cooks and helpers tended the food. Ladies came and went with nibbles and other offerings to the feast and Bev was thinking she might need to get back on her diet after this evening's feast.

Inside JAC the band was set up and Bev noted that young Billy had arrived with Ernie and Mrs. B with all his gear. Bev had a long chat with Mrs. B and Ernie who told her that the car looked like it had run its last mile. Leaving those discussions for another day Bev headed back into JAC to find

Steve and Alice had arrived and wanted to chat before the formalities kicked off.

As ever, Alice had a good turn of phrase when she said.

"Bev, I can see you've got the hook baited we hear that Charlie has taken the bait and you will be under scrutiny tonight girl so be careful how you reel him in" she says. as she admired Bev's red dress and beauty,

"I'm sure I will Alice but I don't really care, let them gossip but the fire is lit and the embers are settling in our emotions, so what will happen will happen but, I'm going to spread myself around tonight to perhaps slow things down a bit."

Smiling at Bev Alice pats her on the shoulder.

"I'm sure the lads here tonight will appreciate your spreading yourself around, especially looking like you do just don't forget who brought you to the dance" says Alice,

"Thanks Alice but this is just an old thing I threw on" says Bev, flicking her hair and giggling as they hug and Alice head toward the stage as Charlie signals to them.

Gathering his daughters, Bev, Amy and Alice around him Charlie gives out instructions.

"Right ladies, here's your donation buckets and note pads, please use your charms to get the buckets filled".

Chat over Charlie takes to the microphone and calls everyone to the hall. After the welcome and the basic arrangements for the night have been explained he announces this year's fund raising is for the school building at Arkeroon Indigenous settlement. He explains the conversion of the old storage sheds into a schoolhouse and medical room for clinics and that a teacher has been found who is willing to come and live on site with her husband.

"So folks, If you have a few bob to spare these lovely ladies would love you to put it in their bucket, If you can help with materials or labour or anything please leave a note with the ladies on their notepads and no they don't want your phone numbers guys, so be generous and lets have a great night dinner will be ready in half an hour and I hope you're hungry as there is plenty to eat. Enjoy the night and thanks for coming."

The ladies pick an area and move off with their buckets. Bev is attracting more than casual attention. Meeting some of the folk she has known at clinics and accidents the comments come thick and fast. Hope this is the new AEROMED uniform Bev and I wouldn't have recognised you, Bev.

Others were more interested in her relationship with Charlie and there were a few who were a bit jealous of this interloper in their territory. As Charlie said he was inundated with pots of stew when Jill passed away. It wasn't until Esmeralda arrived that some of the hopefuls were dissuaded from bringing over food, most of which went to Sam and Jess.

Bev's bucket was filling fast and there were several notes added. She looked across at the other ladies circulating and it looked like they were doing fine also. A couple of the younger guys had asked if she would save a dance for them and she had agreed, thinking this would take some of the heat out of the gossip.

She noted Charlie had a small circle of ladies surrounding him and laughing with the false giggles that women do when they are on the hunt. Bev was not worried as their efforts were so obvious she was sure Charlie could see through the ruse.

Pairing up they went off to circulate around the encampment and chat to people. There was a friendly and sincere atmosphere about the place and she could see a softer side of these hard folk who had hard lives. Amy explained that this was sometime the only respite these folks get amid the hardship of running farms and stations, droughts, floods and poor cattle prices. Bev saw a kind of majesty in these people which made her more determined to dedicate her life and work to these wonderful folk.

Taking the full buckets back to JAC they were ushered into Charlie's office where Steve and he were already counting the booty and reading the notes. Jen was tapping away on the computer at Charlies command. It was then that the band started up. Off you go ladies, that's your que to have a dance with the folks out there.

It wasn't long till Bev was whirling around the floor to modern country rock music, barn dances, oz rock and some traditional stuff with banjos and fiddles appearing out of nowhere. One of the revelations during the rock sets was the booming voice of Sams assistant Trish. She was good and Bev was to learn that she had attended formal classes at the institute of modern music in the city and had travelled as a backup singer to visiting entertainers. During a break, she caught Trish's attention and managed to pry her away from a few would be suitors.

They shared a drink and chatted outside as she explained she was not needed for the next set as it was square dancing stuff. "Trish I'm blown away with your singing voice, what on earth are you doing here and not on the international stage?"

"It's a long story Bev, as you know I was born and raised here, sang in church as a kid, won a local talent quest at a young age and went off to study singing in the city at the institute of modern music. From there I got involved with bands, and did some studio work and backing vocals for visiting artists. I had a manager who ripped me off and left me pregnant. I had the baby adopted in the city, which I still regret but I had no choice and so I returned home here and settled in with my grief.

Showing Bev tattoos which James always remembered.

"I named him before he was taken away. I don't know if he still has the same name but one day I hope he wants to find his birth mum."

"That is so sad Trish, it must have been heartbreaking for you", says Bev.

"Yes, it was but life moves on and I've got lots of friends like you and others that have my back."

Bev puts an arm around her in a sisterly way. A tap on her shoulder causes Bev and Trish to turn around.

"Well, now why aren't you two in there dancing?" It was Sam, hand in hand with a shorter stout man with a manicured beard and a bald spot.

"Sorry were late to the shindig we had a small animal emergency to attend to. Oh Bev, this is my partner Phillip, we are hoping to get married next year, it is all going well. See you two inside and I'm looking forward to your raunchy singing Trish" he says as they leave hand in hand.

Bev was somewhat taken aback at this revelation and Trish noticed her startled look.

"You didn't know he was gay" says Trish.

"Well, no, I didn't, he is such a hunk I often wondered why he didn't have a lady in tow, says Bev.

"The night you stayed at the place when you brought the injured roo in, I had the feeling you had eyes for Sam."

"Well, who wouldn't. I was new in town and the first person I met was a hunk. What a waste," says Bev.

Trish giggles, "that's what most of the ladies in town think also, and don't worry there have been attempts to turn him over to bat for the other side". They laugh and giggle about it as they head back into the dance only to be grabbed by young men and whisked onto the dance floor.

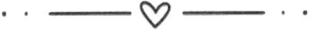

Dance with me

The night was a wonderful mix of music and dancing with different people taking the stage along with Trish, and Charlie who did his Kenny Rogers and Kenny Loggins stuff to great effect and applause. Much to the disappointment of many young guys, Bev had purposefully avoided any slow dances by using the need for a toilet break and other things and not appearing until the slow ones were over. She was reserving that close dance stuff for one man and her pledge to herself to mingle and not fixate on Charlies had been kept.

It was late in the evening when Steve and Tom took to the stage and announced the results of the donations. To the sound of applause Tom gave the good news that they had reached their target and thanked everyone with special mention of those who were contributing materials, equipment and labour. Closing off, Steve announced it was time for the widows hop and three young men with bare upper torsos appeared on stage to the tumultuous cheers and hoots of the crowd. The stock and station auctioneer took to the microphone giving the conditions.

"Right ladies, this is your chance to see out the rest of the evening with one of these hunks, they were certainly well muscled and handsome young men. For those of you who are new to this annual bit of fun the rules are simple. If you want to bid for the company of one of these hunks you need to come and get a paddle from the front of the stage here and after the next short set we will begin the auction.

Bev was a bit taken aback by this sort of meat market thing but Amy always put her distaste into perspective.

"I can see you're a bit of a displeased girlfriend. Let me explain what this is all about, it is a fund raiser for the AEROMED clinics and is quite harmless although it has led to relationships in the past. I bid and won Tom in one of these things."

Bev turned toward Amy with a look of amazement on her face as Amy nodded,

"Sorry Charlie is not up for auction this year as the age groups have changed.

"Hang on Amy, you bid and won Tom in this meat raffle?"

"Yep, best thing I ever did and we are still hanging out for the last dance after all these years. It's harmless fun Bev and you're welcome to bid if you want. It's only till the end of the evening, which isn't far off and after that it's up to the Guy and Gal if they want to take it further. Tom and I did that evening, woohoo!!"

Still aghast Bev says.

"No thanks Amy, I will sit this one out.

"I figured that, I've been watching you and I know who will be getting the last dance with you tonight Go get him girl,", says Amy, slapping Bev on the backside.

"By the way I was only winding you up about Tom and me. We met at a country music festival."

"What am I going to do with you Amy, you had me going there" says Bev hitting Amy playfully on the shoulder.

The auction began with the bidders anxiously holding their paddles. The first young man was led out with a jeweled collar around his neck and a halter rope attached to it. The local stock auctioneer introduced the young man as if he were cattle.

The small clutch of ambitious women of varying ages gathered around the foot of the stage as the auctioneer introduced the first piece of meat.

"Okay here we have a fine young stud bull, good legs and temperament, He has been servicing Heffer in the western regions for some time with great success. the bidding will be in $10 lots so to hold up your paddles when you bid."

The bidding stopped at $200 and the lucky lady claimed her prize leading the young man off the stage to the cheers of the crowd. The next young man was led out with a mock halter around his head and paraded up and down the stage.

"Right ladies, this Jon, a fine young 30-year-old stallion, bred out of Sophia by Jimmy and raised here. He has all his teeth strong forelocks. He has been raised to go all night and thought to have had a good career at stud as far as I'm led to believe. OK, so what am I bid."

The bidding was like a stock auction with the usual fast paced auctioneer chatter and reached a bit over $250 before the hammer dropped and the winning bid announced by paddle number. As the winner led away her prize, it seemed to be all good fun and a bushy way of hooking up but politically correct in the city would find this all horrifying.

The Auction continued in the same way for the last young man and the auctioneers' comments were met with cheers and whoops and the occasional bullshit call. What amazed Bev was that the young men's mothers and fathers were mostly present in the room and watching the auction with big smiles. Maybe that was because they might be getting rid of them with a prospect of gaining a daughter-in-law and grandkids perhaps. Whatever it was it all seemed harmless and good fun.

The band struck up a rousing Kenny Loggins song with Charlie on vocals with Trish. The dance floor was filled with happy people whirling around the floor. Bev had several young guys sweep her around the floor in the next set all hoping for the last dance. It was a fast set and once it was over Trish announced that after a short break, she would be back with the karaoke machine for final set, the cuddle shuffle as she called it. Bev knew what that meant and made a beeline for the toilet with the hope of avoiding the inevitable offers that would come.

Taking her time in the toilet she waited until the music started and skirted around the now darkened room hoping to avoid the young men who had already asked her for a last dance. She was near the door and could see a couple of guys obviously looking for her and starting to make their way over. She was in a dilemma as to what to tell then and hoping that Charlie would be her final partner for the night when she felt a tap on the shoulder. Turning she found herself looking up at Charlies smiling face.

"May I have this dance Maam" he said.

"You most certainly may sir" she replied and fell into his strong arms as Trish sang some beautiful slow love songs.

By the time Trish got to what must be near the end of the set Bev had her head on his chest and was moving slowly to the music. She felt contentment that closeness to a loved one can bring, Charles had his eyes closed and was taking in her perfume and the softness of her body as he nuzzled her hair and sang along softly to the love songs that were so beautifully sung by Trish. No words were spoken or needed between them it was a moment of perfect bliss for them both.

As they shuffled around Bev noticed that two of the auctioned guys were cuddled up to their partners from the auction. Collars removed the young ladies were enjoying their closeness to the muscled chest of their young men and Bev wondered where the other couple had gone to.

Along the way Amy and Tom shuffled past with Amy winking at Bev. Sam and his partner Phil were off in the gloom shuffling away and Bev noticed Jen close by with Billy and Steve and Alice enjoying the dance and music. Even Mrs. B and Ernie were up and doing the cuddle shuffle so it looked like they were an item that called for further discussion.

By the time Trish got to the lovely Bacharach song, the look of love it was clear that Bev was completely involved with Charlie and wanted him as their beautiful music came to an end. Trish then announced we have one more song before we say goodnight. It's a special request from our host Charlie Forest. I hope you like it.

The music started and it wasn't long before Bev realised who it was for. Lady in red was a lovely song and Charlie was looking at her and singing along with the words. The lights had come up a little and a small spotlight was on Charlie and Bev as they moved around the floor for the final dance. It was a moment that would stick with her forever.

The music over the couple stood swaying gently and still in each other's arms.

"Ok Charlie, you can let her go now" says Amy walking up to the mesmerized couple.

Choo Choo

The party was over and most of the cleanup was done when Amy and Bev walked back towards the homestead. Tom, Charlie and Steve headed off in the alligator to check on the various camps and for Steve to leave departure briefing notes for the aviation set. It was quite late but they could see small fires in the distance and the sound of singing and guitars strumming.

Amy turned to Bev as they walked slowly through the homestead gardens.

"Well, how did you enjoy your first Muster Ball girlfriend" she asks.

"What can I say. Apart from the meat auction which I'm still not sure about it was great."

Amy stops her walking and says.

"I need you to understand something about the meat auction. What you don't know is that most of the young men have been going out with the highest bidder for some time. The money they pay is driven on by their girlfriends and parents and it's already forecast who was going to win. The money is returned to the dowry fund of the young ladies and Forest Farms Inc matches it and offers the use of JAC for their reception and a catering pack to help along with the band. In the end it's a kind of mating ritual with a formalized end plan. Last year we had 6 weddings here, four came from the meat auction as you called it."

Bev looks back at Amy,

"I had no idea that was the plan, it just looked a bit crude and obnoxious but now that you've explained it all makes sense. I have a whole new perspective on the mating ritual here now, thanks Amy".

"I think you're well on your way to your own mating ritual sweetheart, and you won't need a meat auction to get there but I'm sure there will be meat in there somewhere." She says.

Punching Amy on the shoulder, Bev laughs and says,

"You are awful, but I like it."

"You do know you've got Charlie's attention Bev, in fact, I hope he stands his little soldier to attention for you before long."

They both giggle as they move towards the homestead with Amy suggesting a nightcap was in order. There was a light on in the kitchen as they entered and Amy switched on the living room lights and headed for the small bar in the corner.

"What will it be sweety, cocktail or beer or?? Hey, Charlie has left his prized bottle of Maker Bourbon out. That's what we will have no arguments."

Bev raises her hands in a mock surrender.

"Okay, let's go for that if you're sure Charlie won't be angry at us getting into his favourite tipple."

"Bev, after your performance tonight he will forgive you anything and he knows better than to challenge me." Both smiling Amy hands Bev the glass and sniffs in the aroma of the bourbon with delight

"Superb, this stuff only comes out on special occasions, I reckon this is one." Says Amy reclining in the lounge chair.

Bev walks over to the mantel piece and looks at the photos.

Amy, I'm curious about something, these pictures show all of you all but who is that guy in the middle?

Walking over, Amy picks up the picture,

"that's Brian Forest, the middle of the 3 sons that Jack and Sarah had. He is no longer with us unfortunately."

"That's sad, what happened to him and did he have a partner or wife and kids" says Bev.

Amy sipping her drink holds up her hand.

"I think you better hold those thoughts for a private discussion with Charlie and Tom. It's a sensitive area and still hurts them both. It's best that they give you the full story and the outcome at a time when your private, relaxed and the mood is right, you will know when, trust me."

Amy went on to discuss the developments of the Stations and the terrible effect Jills death had on Charlie.

"It was one of the worst periods for the family, Tom and I had been busy on developing the farm with Charlie's help. They were so much in love and the two girls completed them as a couple. They did everything together and it was Jills idea to kick off the muster ball.

"As Jill's health declined, we came here more often to help but trying to build our farm and looking after this place was too much and Tom collapsed in the middle of it all which just compounded the situation.

"Tom was whizzed off to hospital and had 3 stents put in. Our wonderful supervisor on the farm helped me keep things going but I couldn't do anything to help Charlie here. By this stage, the girls were at boarding schools in the city so they were only home in the holidays and the occasional long weekend.

"It was clear that Charlie was not coping on his own and his drinking had increased and he became more and more reclusive. Something had to be done as the station was going backwards.

"We had an older couple, Esmeralda and Juan, working for us in the orchards and the bottling area. Tom and I asked if they would like to help look after Charlie until he got back on his feet. The rest is history and they have been almost father and mother to Charlie and Grandparents to the girls ever since.

"Everyone loves them and we have in fact given them shares in the business as an appreciation for their care and concern. I'm sure you will meet them at some stage as it's a given they will want to check you out and approve just in case you look like being part of the family which I must admit is looking more likely after tonight."

They smile warmly at each other as Amy continues.

"You will find Esmerald a matter-of-fact person, great cook and totally devoted to Charlie and vice versa. Tom and I used to come and stay for the occasional weekend to see how Charlie was getting on. At the time Esmeralda and Juan lived here in the homestead whilst Tom and Charlie built them their own place across the way." she says pointing towards a small cottage outside the homestead fence.

"Anyway, one morning when Tom and I got up and headed to get some coffee in the kitchen. Charlie was already up and having breakfast under Esmeralda's charge. As we approached, she held up a finger looking cross she said,

"No more Choo Choo tonight, no more, you sleep OK."

"It had us stumped but we agreed and sat down to Esmeralda's delightful breakfast. Charlie was in a good mood and his demeanor was improving every day.

He smiled at us and said, "You guys sounded like you had fun last night unless there's a steam train in your room. I blushed and Toms mouth hung open. Esmeralda was pouring coffee for us and said,

"No more Choo Choo, need to sleep."

It came home that her polite reference to Choo Choo was based on our lovemaking noises which Charlie had confided in Tom sounded like a steam train going up a hill and then descending. He reckoned I sounded like some kind of high-pitched muffled scream at the pivotal moment. We all laughed whilst Esmeralda in her then broken English smiled,

"No more Choo Choo Ok."

Bev was in fits of laughter with Amy making choo choo noises when Tom and Charlie returned.

"I see Amy's told you about Choo Choo and found my Makers Mark Bourbon" says Charlie smiling.

"Sure, did big fella and its great, can I pour you a glass, Tom, do you want one to?"

"I'm good, says Charlie I've got to fly early in the morning and you know the rules 12 hours bottle to throttle, but I will make myself a cup of tea."

Finishing their drinks and sensing it was time for bed regardless of being tired or not, Amy takes Tom by the arm and leads him to the bedroom winking at Bev and bidding them good night.

CHAPTER 11

———◆◇◆———

Happiness

Lost and Found

C harlie sat close to Bev on the couch as he asked how she found the day and explained he was sorry not to have spent more time with her. Bev put her fingers on his lips and said all I needed was that slow shuffle and you made me very happy with that and I'm beginning to see how life is for you and those wonderful daughters you have.

Charlie moved even closer and it looked like a first kiss was imminent when Tom burst into the room, dragging Amy behind him. Looking at the clipboard in his hand he announces his revelation.

"Charlie, I've got the departure sequence, ah um ah, oh sorry it can wait till morning, I think."

Amy looking apologetic agrees "Yes Tom, you idiot, it can certainly wait till the morning" dragging Tom back up the hallway and making sorry motions to Bev as she went.

"No Choo Choo for him tonight, now get to bed", she says pushing him down the hallway."

However, it was too late, the mood was broken Charlie turned to Bev with an apologetic look on his face as he got up to leave.

"Sorry about that, Bev, I didn't mean to be so forward, it's going to be a big day tomorrow so we best get some sleep" and with that he headed off down the hall to his bedroom.

Bev was speechless and disappointed but figured there would be other opportunities as she followed him down the hall to her room. Sitting on the bed she shed a little tear at the missed kiss and opportunities that might bring.

A gentle tap on her door has her thinking it was probably Amy coming to apologise for Toms insensitivity. Opening the door, she was surprised to see Charlie standing there.

"I am sorry about the conclusion of the evening; big brothers timing was off as always. Perhaps tomorrow we can take up where we left off.

Bev grabbed him by the shirt front and dragged him into the room, locking the door behind him and standing with her back to the door and a naughty smile on her lips.

"Wanna make Choo Choo big boy. I need someone to blow my whistle and you look like the fella to do it" she says as she slowly unbuttons his shirt.

Charlie bends to kiss her and their lips meet in a long passionate kiss. His hands slipping the little red dress off her shoulders, it falls to the floor. His shirt now off Bev slowly kisses his chest and works her way south.

Unbuttoning his trousers it's obvious the large bulge in his undies is ready for action. She gentle reaches inside his underpants and gently rubs his erect shaft whilst Charlie undoes her bra and frees her ample breasts.

He gently fondles her breast as Bev descends to take his shaft in her mouth, gently tickling the top with her tongue and still gently massaging the shaft and caressing his balls intermittently.

Charlie bent over suddenly and gently picked her up in his arms and carried her to the bed laying her down he removed her panties and kicked off his jeans. Now both naked he lavishes kisses on her breast with erect nipples. This was one of Bev's G spots and she loved every lick and suck.

His attention moved down her stomach with gentle kisses until he focused on her waiting vagina. His attention to that area brough Bev to the edge of climax as he licked and sucked her clitoris and gently fingered her vagina.

It was clear this man knew what he was doing and it wasn't long till Bev had an explosive orgasm and shuddered violently at the ecstasy. It had been a long time since she had experienced anything like this.

Charlie moved her fully on the bed and introduced his engorged member to her vagina lips. Not entering her he teased her lips and clitoris with it whilst kissing and sucking her nipples and kissing her lips and neck.

Bev was on the edge of another orgasm as he gently entered her and with a few gentle shoves stopped deep inside her and kissed her passionately. She came with a fury that saw her legs wrapped around his back and her abdominal muscles flexing.

Charles resumed his steady rhythm and kissing her as he went, he sensed she was on the brink of another orgasm and picked up the pace. There was no doubt he timed this perfectly as they came together in a crashing climax. His hot sperm spurting deep inside her seemed to never end as they writhed in pleasure and with her abdominal muscles, squeezing the last amount of sperm and pleasure out of him.

They lay back with her head on his chest.

"I'm sorry he said, it's been a long time since I...

Cutting him off with kisses Bev whispers in his ear

"Don't apologise my beautiful man, you were fantastic, I've never come that often in my life."

After some rest Bev started the next coupling with consideration for Charlie's recovery needs but he was ready for round 2 of Choo Choo and as the night went on, they tried different positions each with the same wonderful results.

Their lust finally sated they lay back in each other's arms and went to sleep around 4am. Bev had found the love and passion she had needed for so long.

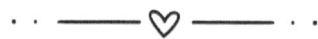

Blissful Rest

With the early morning sun peeking through the blinds, Charlie stood at the end of the bed dressing quietly so as not to disturb Bev. He watched her sleeping and knew he was in love with this woman and hoped the feelings were mutual.

Her hair spilled sensuously over the white pillow and her slightly tanned skin was a contrast to the white sheets. Her looks and perfectly formed body delighted him and raised thoughts about waking her up for a morning session but he had lots of stuff to do today so he put the thought aside for later.

There was still that feeling of guilt like he was cheating on Jill but Tom had reminded him of her words in the final days of her fight for life when she held his hand asking him to look after their girls and to be happy.

Now he understood what that meant and this beautiful lady had shown her the way to that happiness. He dreamed last night that Jill came to him and repeated the words be happy, she is good for you. Happy with his thoughts he quietly closed the door as he left meeting Amy in the Hallway with a knowing smile on her face as she passed.

The door closing woke Bev to find she was alone and her thoughts went instantly to the possibility of it being a one-night stand. Her past experiences and paranoia triggered her thinking about it as she showered and dressed and headed to the kitchen for breakfast. Her fears were pointless as she was kissed and hugged wholeheartedly by Charlie in front of Tom and Amy in a way that says we are one.

"I guess there was some Choo Chooing last night guys, did you blow your whistles" she says looking over the top of her sunglasses as they laughed and sat down for breakfast.

"Big day today folks Charlie, do you want to run through what's on for Bev and Amys sake?" says Tom.

Sure, I'm flying out to check on the strip at Lake Edward and I thought Bev might like to come for the ride." says Charlie.

"Like she wouldn't" said Amy winking at Bev.

Continuing Charlie points to the clipboard on the table,

"Tom, I think you and Steve should do the flight ops stuff and briefing and I will do the briefing for those flying to the strip at the lake when I get back.

"It's early so I don't imagine anyone will want to leave yet but just in case lets drive the flight line. Jen is coming out with us and staying in the boathouse overnight so she can get an early start with her camera the next day.

"I think Billy will likely drive out there later today and I know Steve and Alice are also planning to head there around lunch time so she won't be on her own tonight. Right, let's get to it, Bev can you grab that thermos and the Esky and chuck them into the alligator whilst I go over the departures with Tom."

"Ever the gent, welcome to the female pack horse party girl-friend. says Amy,

Charlie looks up to see Bev smiling at him.

"It okay, you're busy and I'm happy to help. she says, giving him a peck on the cheek as she leaves.

LITTLE YELLOW BIRD

A short time later the foursome pulls up outside Charlie's hanger to find Jen pulling the Robinson out with the small tractor. Amy and Bev unloaded the stuff, going out to the lake and helping Jen pack it into the helicopter carefully.

"That's a whole lot of stuff for today" says Bev.

"Not really Dad wants to clean up the strip and is meeting one of the locals who will be there to help as needs be. Weight and balance wise with the three of us he will be near the limit but its fine as there is a good margin in the load weights." Says Jen

Bev is dazzled by Jen's aviation knowledge as Charlie and Tom come back dropping Charlie off to do discuss the Lake Edward strip preparation with fellow pilots. Amy in the Alligator with Tom heads back to Homestead.

Charlie returns from his discussions.

"OK ladies let's get out of here.

Jen had taken the front left seat next to dad so she could get a couple of hours into her logbook under dad's careful guidance as they flew off to the lake. Their arrival at the small grass strip was uneventful with Bev helping Jen get the gear to the boatshed and set up the room for her.

Charlie was in conversation with a guy on a tractor who was preparing to mow and clear the grass strip. They finished their individual tasks and were soon back in the air and heading back to the homestead with Jen waving from the ground. Charlie explained the need to clear the strip and make sure there were no soft spots and the neighbor had it all in hand with his team clearing the threshold and grading the hard stand area as well as checking the tie down points.

They were soon back at Forest Station and set the helicopter down near the hangar which was now full of people. Charlie explained that this was the departure briefing and I'm going to brief them on the airstrip at the lake. Stick around I have something I want to show once Steve and Tom get this lot out of here.

Tom and Steve were busy addressing the group of people about the departure requirements and the order of departure by call sign with the pilots scribbling everything down including a couple of radio frequencies. Steve will be up in the loft calling the shots so keep your ears and eyes open remember it's a see and be seen procedure. Any questions. The silence meant there was none.

Right lets go to it and wait for those start up responses. Those staying on or heading out to the lake tomorrow, Charlie will give you a briefing. With that a couple of pilots and there folk left whilst Steve climbed the ladder to the loft and balcony on top of the hanger overlooking the airfield. Once finished Charlie invites Bev to climb the ladder and watch Steve at work.

It was amazing to see the precision of it all at the relatively re-mote airstrip. Charlie explained that an accident about 5 years ago brought all this under scrutiny by the aviation authority. Fortunately, no one was badly injured but the wreck of one of the Aircrafts is still out there he says pointing to a tail sticking out of some swampy brush.

Bev was curious and asked what happened. Charlie explained that the Aircraft out in the swampy ground was taking off when another decided to taxi. That Aircraft out there had no choice but to try and hop over the other one and he nearly made it but his under carriage struck the wing of the other Aircraft and veered off to the swampy ground landing heavily whilst the other Aircrafts hit the fence. Everyone walked away but it could have been worse.

The Aircraft out there was considered not worth recovering by the insurers so with the owner's permission we stripped parts off it including its radio sets that Steve is using now.

We keep the wreck there as a reminder to others of what can happen and why we are a bit tough on them.

"Come on, I've got something to show you," says Charlie helping her down the ladder and heading off to the back of the hanger through a large door into another smaller hangar.

Sitting in the middle of the hangar was a small yellow high winged Aircraft with a tail wheel.

"I wanted to show you this and to offer you lessons to fly it or rather share flying it with Jen who is doing solo checks in it. This is probably the simplest Aircraft in the air, it's a piper cub and I've added the big balloon tyres. Come take a look and hop in if you want."

Bev was a little dumbstruck and could only follow Charlie to the pretty little Aircraft. As, they walked over Charlie explained that it was Jills Aircraft and she flew it often during muster and could land it on a sixpence or drop sandwiches to the guys. Apart from Jen and probably Annie in due course it sits here. When Jen heads off to Uni and Annie goes back to boarding school it will sit here doing nothing. I have an instructor rating and I thought we could spend some time together teaching you to fly her.

"Jump in, it's flown from the back seat as you will learn, there's very few instruments and the stick and rudder controls are all connected by wire." he says.

Sitting in the rear seat Bev was at once in love with this little bird. Reaching out she grabbed Charlie's face and kissed him.

"You're a beautiful man but the Aircraft must have memories for you and I don't want to get in the way of those or your girls use of their Mums Aircraft."

OK, I hear what you say but if you don't use it, I will likely sell it as I can't justify having it just sitting here. If you learn to fly it will mean you can fly yourself around the station and help me and take it back to town and our hangar their which would be a great help for services and for the girls to grab and fly out to the Homestead when they come home from Uni and school. So, you see my offer has more than sentiment attached to it." said Charlie.

Kissing him again she continues holding his face and says,

"Well, if you're sure then I would love to learn to fly under your teaching in this wonderful little Aircraft." Kissing him again she pulls back with a disappointed look on her face.

"There one problem, there's not enough room for choo choo".

Charlie hugs her and kisses her as he lifts her out of the seat.

"You're right but I know a place nearby where train operations are allowed and it's comfortable," he says leading her toward a little office on the side of the hangar.

An hour later, with a lot of choo chooing done they straighten their clothing and head out through different doors back to the homestead. Bev exited through the door they came in through and back into the main JAC room where the party and dance had been.

Hearing woos woo train noises from behind her Bev turns to see Amy coming out of Charlies office with an arm full of books. Blushing brightly Bev asks,

"Were you listening in Amy?"

"No sweety, but the wall between the two hangars is thin and the workshop only has a mess roof to keep the birds out. It also echoes in there; I know because Tom and I have used it. Got any splinters in your butt." They both giggle.

"No, we used the lounge. says Bev.

"Oh, ok then, but you may have fleas as that was the dogs favourite spot when the hangar was active. Not a good look scratching your nether regions at lunch girlfriend. but I suppose you can scratch each other's at the dinner table." says Amy frowning,

Both women have a fit of giggles like a pair of naughty students as they walk out of the big doors on JAC. Coming across from the dormitory direction Alice stops them saying, what are you two giggling about as if I don't know as she winks at Bev.

Trying to make some sense of the encounter, Bev says.

"He was just showing me his little yellow Aircraft and...

Alice interrupts her, holding her hand and staring questioningly at Bev.

"Oh, so that's what he is calling it these days. Did you help him put his little yellow Aircraft in your hangar sweety?" she says?

They all laughed as Bev smiled and said with a naughty look.

"I might have!" with a demure grin on her face.

"So apart from that what was it he wanted to show you" asked Alice.

Bev explains the discussions about her learning to fly in the little Aircraft and how they were planning to stay here tonight and fly out in it to the lake tomorrow, she went on to explain that they may even fly back to town on Monday so I can get some stick and rudder time he said.

Amy, ever the joker couldn't resist a pun,

"In these parts' girlfriend that's shorthand for cock and udder time after the flying bit.

"The three giggle and laugh as they head along the path until Alice grabs Bev's arm pulling her up.

"You do know what this means Bev she says with an earnest look on her face, this man is getting serious, he has had a few other women out here before."

Amy is quick to put her thoughts in "You mean the sperm spittoons; there were some doozies. Remember the blonde unit with the huge tits. She could breast feed all the poddy calves from those babies" giggling again at Amy's humour sets them off again.

Composing herself, Alice continues.

"Some of those women feigned interest in the Cub but none were allowed near it let alone sit in it or have him offer to teach them to fly in it. I think you've hook him sweety but move slowly there are still ghost attached to that Aircraft."

"I'm aware of that Alice, in fact I mentioned that and declined his offer based on it being Jills Aircraft and I wouldn't want to cut across any emotional ties. He explained that after Jen completes her solos and sits her license test in the next couple of weeks she will be heading to university for some time and Annie will be heading back to boarding school, so after the holidays the Aircraft was likely going to be sold as it's unlikely to be used again for some time. There was plenty of interest in the little Aircraft and he would have no problem selling it. But he felt if it could be kept active between Jens trips home it would be worth keeping. He knew I was considering learning after he talked with Brad and so it all seemed to fit."

"Not be too bad a way to get some stick and rudder time under Charlie I suspect" says Amy. More laughter and nods of agreement

"So, you're coming out to the lake," asks Alice. "

"Yep, Charlie and I plan fly out after we get rid of you."

"Good, time to get on girls" says Amy, "Tom will be chaffing at the bit to get off to the lake". Walking away Amy looks over her shoulder making train noises and Woo Woo Woo sounds.

"What's that all about" asks Alice?

"I will let Amy explain to you someday, it's a private joke we have." says Bev.

"I think I get it" and I'm happy for you both. Everyone commented on what a lovely couple you made last night and we all think you are so right for each other, just don't rush it sweety, he is still delicate inside despite the hard exterior, get to know him." says Alice gently holding Bev's shoulders and looking deep into her eyes.

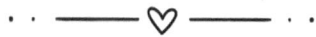

The Lake

The mid-day sun shone through the blinds in the Kitchen. Bev headed for the shower to freshen up and was not surprised when Charlie joined her in the shower. Gently rubbing bodywash over her body and kissing her neck, it was clear to Bev where this was going.

He lifted her against the shower wall and entered her with an urgency she had not seen before. The love making was abrupt and energetic with both reaching a climax at the same time shuddering and sinking to the floor under the still running shower.

"Guess we need another shower now sweetheart" says Charlie.

"Oh, I don't know, we've been wasting water you know but I couldn't reach the tap" says Bev with a devilish smile on her face.

"Fuck the water waste my lovely" says Charlie smiling as he turns off the tap. Picks her wet body up and carries her to the bed where they slowly caressed and cuddled until she took Charlie's half erection in her mouth until he was ready. The love making was slow and prolonged with her coming twice before Charlie unloaded in her willing vagina.

"Now we need another shower," says Charlie,

"You go first and I will make the bed but it will need clean sheets later after that last workout, but we better get going if we are going to the lake. Says Charlie smirking to himself.

With a knowing smile and flick of her damp hair she heads for the shower, smiling over her shoulder she says,

"Want to come and scrub my back again big boy?"

"You know what happens If I say yes, my temptress" says Charlie.

"Exactly" says Bev with a lascivious grin on her face as she swings her naked hips as she heads to the bathroom.

"Umm! Tempting though it is Maam, but I need some strength for flying today so get in there and wash up, oh, and spare the water this time." He says chasing her playfully into the bathroom with a tap on her naked backside.

"Yes Sir," Bev's responded looking around the bathroom with a sexy smile as she closed the door and thinking I could take more of this.

Sometime later after she had dressed and whilst Charlie showered and shaved, she headed to the kitchen to make sandwiches for them.

Taking the scene in Charlie says,

"I hope she cooks as well as she fucks."

The words took Bev by surprise until she turned around and saw this wonderful man smiling from ear to ear. Walking over slowly and seductively to Charlie she puts her arms around his neck.

"Lunch first and then I will give you another ride cowboy." They kiss and pull apart laughing at the scene they had just played which reminded them both of a cowboy western with erotic scenes.

Lunch over even the washing up was a chance to cuddle and kiss but time was marching on and they wanted to get the cub out and clean up before the flight to the lake.

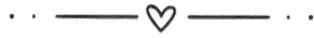

The little yellow bird

There was some playful hosing whilst cleaning the little yellow Aircraft and it wasn't long till Charlie finished a preflight check and had Bev sitting in the back seat for her first flight whilst he swung the prop by hand. With their headphones on, Charlie had taken her through the starting procedure and the very basic instrument as well as the general takeoff and flying requirement.

The engine started after a few swings and Charlie headed for the front seat which he said would be Bev's on the way back. As he went through the taxi and takeoff checks he had Bev repeat them and read off the little card in the side pocket.

Lining up on the airstrip he opened the throttle and talked to Bev about what he was doing and suggested she keep he hand lightly on the stick and her feet on the pedals so she could feel the Aircraft. In a surprisingly short time, they were airborne and climbing into the afternoon sun. At about 2000 feet Charlie headed the little bird toward the lake and handed the stick over to Bev.

She did some turns and climbs and other little maneuvers as they headed out. She loved this little bird and when Charlie suggests they drop the side window things she was sold as the air rushed in and gave her a real sensation of flying.

No wonder Jill loved this thing. It was slow but very maneuverable, it seemed simple to fly and when Charlie handed over the controls and told her to steer a certain course. Bev was beside herself with joy and felt she had found a niche she would love as well as the lovely man she had found.

They reached the lake in due course and Charlie took over the doing a low pass over the camp area and the grass strip before setting her down gently with a little bounce from the balloon tyres as she settled on the grass and they taxied up to the ramp area set aside for the numerous aircraft visiting for the return of the bird festival. Amy and Tom were the first to greet them asking her how she liked flying the Cub whilst Tom and Charlie headed off to see the rest of the family and friends gathered nearby. Bev only had a couple of words for the experience and said,

"I'm in love with the little bird and that man Amy, we had the most wonderful night together and before you ask, no Choo Choo, well not until this morning anyway."

Bev went on to explain the exorcism of ghosts and demons of the past being put to rest and that she had slept in Charlie's bed with him.

Amy hugged her and said,

"Welcome to the family sweety. We are going to have so much fun together and I'm very happy for you both. I've not seen Charlie's face look that happy for a long time. You do understand that Charlies room has been locked since Jill died so you really did lay some ghosts to rest and I'm sure if Jill is looking down, she would be happy to."

More cuddles and a few little tears later and they headed off to the boathouse to catch up with everyone.

The afternoon flew by with Jen taking Bev out in the floating hide to photograph the various birds. They swam in the separated area with Charlie and others splashing about happily. It was lucky she remembered to bring her modest one-piece swimsuit in lieu of the skimpy thing Amy offered.

"Here you go girl, you got it so show it she had said" with a sly giggle when she first presented it to her on their shopping spree.

Around 3pm Charlie came over and said they should think about leaving after he had taken Jen up to do her aerial photography thing. Concerns about an approaching storm had others worried and there were movements among the pilots to prepare their Aircraft for takeoff or tie down.

Flying Training Intensifies

This time Bev had the front seat.

Charlie put his hand on her shoulder and said,

"You can do this just relax and follow what I taught you and I will be right here to take over if I see you're having any trouble".

Speaking slowly and directly he guided her through the take-off and she amazed herself when they lifted into the air a little bit off the centre line but wings level and with a steady rate of climb.

"You got this, now look outside and make left turn and fly a heading of 090."

Remembering where the compass was, she banked left remembering to use a little rudder as Charlie had shown her and with just a little over correction she had the Aircraft on the heading.

"Watch your altitude and keep 2000 ft." said Charlie patting her on the shoulder.

Finding the altimeter, she saw she was passing 1700ft with a slow rate of climb.

"Watch your attitude we don't want to stall," said Charlie.

She remembered his chat about the angle of attack as she put the nose down slightly.

Making small corrections she came up to 2000 feet and was heading 090.

"On course and altitude Captain" she said.

"Right, now pull the power back a little and we can cruise home."

Bev was beside herself; this was real flying as compared to the high-altitude pressurized King Air and others she had flown in with Brad. Charlie lowered the side curtains and the rush of air was even more exhilarating. As they flew on Charlie pointed out his bore pumps, the occasional emu or kangaroo herd.

Life couldn't get any better she thought and came then daunting task to land. She was a bit nervous and Charlie felt it as he touched her tense shoulders and walked her through the procedure for landing.

She practiced the downwind, base and final legs of a typical approach but did a go round.

"Ok Maam, this is the real one, make your all stations radio call for downwind and check the pattern for other Aircrafts."

Charlie made sure she flew an extended downwind leg before turning base, then guided her on final as she lost altitude but kept direction. His soft unhurried tones kept her calm and in control as the little Aircraft came down on the strip when Charlie told her to flare and close the throttle.

The little bird settled down on the grass strip and tracked along the center of the strip. Patting her on her shoulder Charlie says,

"There you go, first takeoff and landing in the cub. I think a few more lessons and we will have you soloing in no time."

She was still shaking when they shut down the engine outside the hangar. It couldn't get any better, she thought but she needed a drink.

Putting the little bird away with a big dust cover over the Aircraft they headed for the homestead leaving the hangar main door open for Tom and Amy to put their Cessna in when they returned.

Hand in hand they headed back as the sound of an Aircraft motor could be heard in the distance.

"I don't think we have time for Choo Choo sweetheart, Ithat will be Tom and Amy arriving so let's get some drinks sorted for them" said tom nuzzling Bev's neck.

It wasn't long before Tom and Amy were sitting together enjoying a drink and recalling the day and Bev's introduction to flying that Charlie said he was most impressed with.

TIME FOR LOVE

Dinner over and rain setting in outside, the four friends sat having coffee and discussing the fund raising and Bev's friend Mary for some time until the conversation turned to cattle prices and crop issues, which was generally the time for the ladies to head off to bed.

Walking up the long hall with Amy Charles reminds her which room to go to as a kind of statement that she is with me now. Amy smiled knowingly and whispered,

"Quiet choo choo tonight please Bev as we are right next door sweety. Ok" says Amy tapping Bev on her arm,

"I will bite the pillow if that helps" says Bev with the girlish giggles noticed in the lounge room by the men who smiled at each other. Tom saying,

"She is a delight brother and I'm so happy to see what she has brought into your life again. After you drop her back to town tomorrow I suggest we run over the school funding plans and the cattle and crop prices. Now I think you need to go and love that women don't you."

"I certainly do big brother, I certainly do." As he rose to head to the bedroom.

CHAPTER 12

———◆O◆———

Nature Strikes Back

The Flood

C harlie's phone rang unexpectedly and it was Jen.

"Hi Jen, getting late you had a good day out there", says Charlie as he listens intently sitting walking back to the lounge room.

"Ok, Ok stay on the line for a minute whilst I talk to Uncle Tom."

Charlie explains the storm hit them badly out there and the lake has flooded the campsites and the airstrip. They can't get out as the access road is underwater. Putting the phone on speaker mode Charlie asks.

"What's happening with the weir and the sluice valves?" Listening intently, he says,

"What! They're locked and the weir is blocked by logs".

Tom jumps in,

"I know what this is and we will fix it later but for now it's dark and we need to get everyone out, how many are we talking about "he says.

"There are about 12 people, which includes 3 kids under 12.and 2 aircraft stuck here as well." Having overheard the discussions, the ladies come back to the lounge room,

Tom finishes his discussion with Jen telling her to hang in there and try to find higher ground, we will come out in the Robinson and get you all moved."

Tom confronts the small group and takes charge.

"Ok guys we have a mission on our hands. Amy, you know the locals near the intersection of Lake Road and the southern highway, can you call them and see if they can get some vehicles out there and warn them about trying to go to the lake and that we will try and move the stranded folk to the road.

"Bev, can you get hold of AeroMed duty staff and let them know what we are doing and ask them to get hold of the police and the Ambo's in case we need some medical help. Charlie and I will get the Robinson ready to fly and could you ladies knock up some Thermos flasks of coffee and throw some leftover food into the small Esky for us?

"Charlie, we will fly out in the R4 and you can leave me there with the tools etc. and start moving folks back to the crossroads. I think Jen can set up a flare point or torch for you. I will call her when we are airborne."

It wasn't long before they were airborne in the dark leaving the hangar lights and others on to help with their return, Charlie was concerned about setting the Robinson down in the flooded area and suggested he do a low hover so Tom can find an area where he can set down with some certainty of getting off again.

Arriving at the lake torches highlighted areas Charlie carefully entered a low hover with water flying everywhere from his prop was, Tom grabbed the Esky and tool bag and jumped down into the knee-high water and headed towards the torches, whilst Charlies backed off and circled the area and the weir.

Seeing the carefully placed logs across the weir and the fact that the sluice valves were locked shut meant it was a deliberate act and he had a pretty good idea who had done it.

Circling back Tom called him and pointed his high beam torch toward him from a small hill about 200 m from the boathouse. Setting the Robinson down but keeping the engine running, he tells Tom about the logs at the weir and that opening the sluice valves is the only thing to do. In the distance Jen is wading through the water with a little child on her shoulders and lady with 2 older kids behind her. Putting them in the chopper and making them secure she says, that's your first load Dad as she closes the door and heads back to the boathouse.

It was a relatively quick trip to the junction and the number of headlights that had formed a circle in the nearby layby area showed Charlie where to land. His passengers unloaded into the waiting arms of the people with blankets and warm drinks he heads back to the lake. The process went on until all the stranded folk were deposited at the junction with the police and ambulance people when they arrived. His final trip back was to pick up Tom and Jen and head back to the Homestead. On the flight back they discussed the sluice valves and the weir.

It was clearly an Abercrombie thing which they had been planning and promising to do for years to increase the backup water for their properties to the north of the Lake. Jen was concerned about the low nesting birds and thought many would have lost their nests and chicks.

It was after midnight before they were back at the homestead and the chopper safely back in the hangar. They made their way back to the house to be greeted by warm drinks and hugs.

Tom was concerned about the logs on the weir and they discussed asking a local if he could bring his D9 Caterpillar out with some chains to drag the logs out. Jen said she had already taken several photos of the weir and sluice valve along with scenes of the flash flooding and the stranded Aircrafts and cars. They agreed they should take copies to the regional authorities with lists of the people that were stranded.

It was clear the three rescuers were dog tired, and it wasn't long before they headed off to take a shower and get some sleep. Amy and Bev did a quick clean-up before heading off and saying good night to each other.

Charlie was sprawled out on the bed with a towel around him and fast asleep. Bev lovingly took the rug from the end of the bed and covered him up kissing her fingertips and touching the top of his head. She realised how tired she was and what big day it had been. Rather than disturb her beautiful man she undressed down to her under clothes and gently lay on the bed next him pulling the sheet over her.

Drifting off to sleep she had a warm sense of belonging and growing love for the man beside her and his family. Things had certainly changed in her life but she still had the feeling it was all too good to be true.

Vandalism

The morning was bright and sunny when they awoke after a long sleep. Tom and Charlie had overslept and when they finally got up it was after 9am. Amy, Bev and Jen slept on and were only woken up by the sounds of the men talking in the kitchen and tools rattling.

It became clear that none of them had remembered to charge their phones and the storm had apparently knocked out the land lines somewhere. Power was also off and the generators had not cut in for some reason. The men were preparing to sort out the generator when the three ladies appeared bleary eyed asking what was going on.

Tom filled in the gaps whilst Charlie gathered more tools. It seems the power had gone out in the storm and the generator was not working, Charlie was going to find some small portable gensets they used on the muster camps whilst Tom had a crack at the main backup diesel generator. Amy and Bev set about tidying up and working out how they might prepare some breakfast without power whilst having a glass of orange juice.

Luckily, the stove was fed on bottled gas, so they set about making bacon and eggs and slicing up some fruit. Toast was out of the question until Jen showed them a trick that Annie taught her using a waffle iron.

It wasn't long before Tom was back and sitting down to the hastily prepared breakfast with the news that a fuel hose had been cut on the generator and the whole shed was flooded with diesel fuel. The large tank also had numerous holes punched in it. There was no way to repair it and it would likely mean a new tank, but they might be able to borrow a portable one from a neighbour temporarily.

Charlies' news was no better when he joined the table, all the small gensets were damaged beyond repair and farm vehicles and tractor tyres slashed and ignition key holes ripped out.

Discussions followed about who would have done this, but as Tom put it, it looked like the work of either activists or the Abercrombie's but the lake flooding problem looked more like the Abercrombie's work. A lock at the weir with ABER marked on it still wouldn't be enough to prove who put the locks on the sluice valves.

Charlie spoke in quiet but direct terms.

"We better get organised in case they come back, Tom, can you take Bev and Jen back to town in the Cessna."

Jen was adamant that she wanted to stay and help as was Bev, but Charlie was having none of it.

"Listen to me you two. There is nothing you can do here and in fact you will worry me more if you are here as I don't know what we are facing here. Also, Bev you've got a Clinic mission to do. Jen, you can hang at AeroMed base until Alice and Steve get back. In the interim, whilst you're there you could print out some of your photographs you took but before you go take some photos of the diesel generator and the vehicles etc." he said in commanding voice.

"That's sensible ladies, as Charlie says your just going to add to his worries if you stay here and Jen, I could use your help with those pictures and the list of names before I go to see the authorities.

"I will preflight the Cessna whilst Charlie locks up as much as he can and opens the gun locker." added Tom putting an arm around Jen with a kind of finality that meant the discussion was over.

"The gun locker, do you think it will come to that" says Amy,

Holding her by the shoulders Tom could see the fear in her eyes. "No, I don't think we are in for a gunfight but its best to be prepared."

Charlie returns with a 3030 rifle, shotgun and a 22 rifle and with Toms help they begin putting the bolts back in the rifles and checking the shotgun and the boxes of ammunition. Handing the 22 to Amy Tom smiles and says,

"Just in case OK" as he and Charlie leave

Guns unslung by their side, Tom and Charlie head to the hangar whilst Amy and Jen head off to photograph things. Bev busied herself in the kitchen making up some cold meat sandwiches and more juice packs for Charlie. Amy and Jen were the first to return, Amy looking like Annie Oakley with the rifle across her chest facing down.

"I see you've got Charlie's siege rations sorted sergeant Bev."

Smiling and holding up small tube of water Bev explains

"I had a thought whilst you were gone, I want to test a sample of the tap water when I get back to town, you never know if that's been tampered with so Charlie should stick to juice for now."

Coming through the door Charlie questions

"Whose got to stick to juice," says Charlie as they enter the room.

Holding up the tube Bev restates her fears.

"I figured that if they could do so much obvious damage, they might have fiddled with the water tank or busted the filtration system. It won't take me long to test it back in town but till I give all clear big fella, drink this stuff only right."

"Yes, Maam" says Charlie giving her a cuddle.

So, we all set to go, girls, I've checked the Cessna and it looks fine as does the Piper so I figure the damage was done whilst we were at the Lake with both those birds" say Tom.

"That makes sense, but the Robinson was here and we used it last night and I didn't give that a thought. I will walk over with you and check it out just in case." says Charlie.

Damaged helicopter

Whilst the ladies loaded up Tom and Charlie went over the Robinson and found a small pool of fluid on the hangar floor. A closer examination revealed a series of pin holes punched in a main line. It was very subtle but dangerous as the hose could have burst in flight with horrendous outcomes given the mercy flights, as well as Tom and Jens return to the homestead.

Jen came over to announce they were all loaded and ready and asked what they had found. Pointing to the small puddle on the floor no words were needed.

"I will get my camera" she says without being asked.

Charlie waved goodbye to the group around mid-morning and resumed his vigil in the JAC office having his cameras back up and running. Tom had promised to try and contact Fred and Jim the neighbors on his CB radio in the Cessna once he was airborne to see if they could come over to help Charlie.

In the meantime, Charlie set about fixing what he could of the solar powered stuff in his office and remembered there was an auto record on some of his boundary cameras that Jen had asked to be installed so she could track the wildlife visitors.

Perhaps they may have recorded something he thought as he sipped his orange juice and hoped the solar batteries had enough charge to run the screens as he began scanning back slowly through the recordings for the last 48 hours.

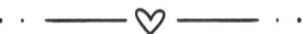

Back in town

Sometime later Tom had set the little Cessna down on the main runway in town and taxied to the Forests hangar. Leaving the Aircraft outside he went into the hangar to make a few calls and charged his mobile phone whilst the three ladies headed over to the AeroMed buildings.

The place was buzzing with activity and a knowing smile from the receptionist and a few of the paramedics told Bev that her relationship with Charlie was no longer a secret. Ascending the stairs to the Ops room they found Steve and Dr Web in deep discussion. Amy made her way to the photocopier whilst Jen sat down at a computer to download her photos.

What's happening, says Bev noting the big smiles on both Steve and Dr Webs' faces.

Maybe you can tell us BEBE the belle of the ball.

Oh, that she says, okay yes, I think Charlie and I are an item but it's still early days.

Dr Web was quick to put his arm around her shoulder. He knew more about her depression and feeling of worthlessness than anyone having treated her symptoms since she arrived and asked for a strong medication. Whispering in her ear he says,

"I'm so very pleased you've found someone, and he is one of the best. I guess you won't be needing that prescription again".

With a tear in the corner of her eye, she smiled at the kindly old doctor who had helped her so much to overcome the trauma of the city. Nodding as she hugged him, she felt very much a part of a bigger team and a community.

The water evaluated ok and she managed to call Charlie and let him know. The neighbors had rallied round and were helping Charlie repair what they could. Tom ordered a new diesel tank and arranged for Charlies engineers to borrow a temporary and get some new hoses for Tom and Ernie to take out on their return to the Homestead. Several sets of tyres were ordered and some temporary used ones were put in the Cessna.

Later that day Bev was relieved from the clinic mission and was able to return to the talk Tom into taking her out to the Homestead despite his and Charlies protests.

"I don't care I want to be with Charlie regardless of the issues" she said as she loaded some easy food stuffs she had picked up in town, into the Cessna.

CHAPTER 13

Love Found

Committment

Tom, Ernie and Bev arrived at the Homestead with a greeting from Charlie standing outside the hangar with a rifle slung across his chest and looking like Wyatt Earp and motioning then not to park in the usual place.

Running to him she takes Charlie's face in her hand's tears streaming down her chin.

"I'm so glad you're ok and how is it all going, any trouble?"

With his arms around her he looked deep into her eyes.

"Nothing more has happened sweetheart and I'm glad you're here. Got any food I'm starving and the crew could do with a feed as well."

Tom came over and asked why the changing of parking spot for the Cessna and Charlie explained that the front of the hangar had been doused in petrol and there were several bullet holes on the façade.

"It looks like we might have interrupted their little game when we came back. We hosed down as much of the fuel as we could but there's still some in the dirt and the last thing I wanted was to have the Cessna catch fire."

"Good thinking Charlie, any luck with the power"

"it's very interesting. One of the guys rode his trail bike down the line from the Homestead to the main junction where the power poles divide off to us and the other properties down the side road. Our mains pole was sawed down along with 2 others so that's why the power was out. It also killed a couple of calf's who got tangled up and electrocuted."

"That's terrible news. Any chance of fixing the poles," said Tom.

"Not at this stage until the power company turns off the live end of the feed. We put up some cattle barriers around the damage and we should be back up in a week or so.

"Also, the LPG main tank had been damaged so we can't use the stove I've ordered a new on from town which should be here tomorrow" says Charlie crossing his fingers.

Holding hands, he leads Bev back to the homestead as Tom and Ernie load up a trolley with the tyres and food Bev had brought with her.

"Sweetie, I think we should use the JAC Barbeque to get some stuff cooking before it gets too dark. I've got to help Tom and Ernie with the tyres and see if we can get the big generator running if you're okay doing the cooking," said Charlie.

Nodding she went on to fire up the gas fired barbeque and got some food off the trolley as it passed. Tom also suggested there should be some steaks in the freezer that should be ok as it's not been opened. It was like old times at home when she was a kid and had prepared the barbecue.

with her father and mother

The Commitment

Later that evening after everyone had something to eat. Tom and Ernie announced they had managed to get the generator started with the help of a loaned portable tank and some temporary fuel hoses fitted. Charlie had also managed to get some good footage of the vandals who were on trailbikes and quite heavily armed.

Watching the footage on Charlie's laptop, Tom commented that it looks like the sound of the chopper scared them off and they hid in the marsh land until we went inside.

"That explains why we still had power before going to bed," said Charlie.

"I'm guessing they waited out there until all was quiet and headed down the fence line to damage the power poles," said Tom.

"I'm going to send the images to the police officers in town. Can you check out the bikes when you go back as they look a bit high end for muster bikes. Jen might be able to clear the images up before we take those to the police" said Charlie yawning.

Tom and Ernie headed off to the workers' accommodation with the others so they could be close to the generator and take watches checking the airfield and the perimeter during the night just in case the vandals wanted a second go.

Bev and Charlie sat quietly in the dim light of a couple of kerosene lamps with her head on his shoulder. She looked up at Charlies tired face and gently stroked his chin.

"I want you to know regardless of where our relationship is heading, I will always be there for you when you need me. "She said kissing Charlie who is looking deep into her eyes.

She was filled with emotion and the tears just came from nowhere and spilled down her cheek. Gently wiping the tears away from her eyes, Charlie held her close and said.

"I think we best head off to bed as we have a big day tomorrow. Holding her hand they walked down the long corridor, pausing at Bev's room as she looked to lead him inside.

"Not tonight sweet lady, this way he says leading her on to his room." Bev's mind was running back to comments about the use of this room and she hoped Jills ghost would be smiling on them now.

This was a symbolic gesture as no one had slept in that room but him as it was his a Jills special place and he kept it locked. Leading her inside he embraced her and they shared a deep and emotional kiss.

They undressed each other and climbed into bed and cuddled till they fell asleep. There was no sex that night as the deep meanings and emotions swept over them both. Words or sex would have ruined the feeling that ran between them that night and it seemed certain that when they woke, they would be different people but deeply committed to each other and the love they now shared.

Bev had found the happiness she craved in this man's arms. Her friend Mary would soon be coming to visit and she couldn't wait to introduce Charlie to her.

There were still ghosts to be exorcised but the love between them was now so strong she was sure they would soon be put to rest. Reflecting on the past few days she could not believe she was here lying next to this beautiful, caring man in this wonderful place.

Where this romance would lead was still uncertain but she was happy to take it slowly and let it develop. For now, she had found love and that was enough for now she thought as she cuddled into Charlies Chest and felt his heartbeat and his breathing slow and soft on her ear.

Nothing could be better than finding the love she never thought she would in this remote part of the world. She bent over and gently kissed Charlie on the cheek and thought how lucky she was. Enjoying the moment, she drifted off to sleep happy in her newfound world of love and excitement.

The End

or is it?

About the Author

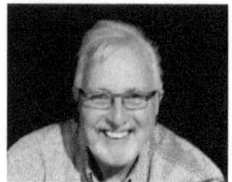

Thor Wesenlund

Thor is an Australian born author from a Norwegian father and Irish mother. Thor has worked in script editing and short stories part time since 1979. His early life in the Navy as a submariner and later as an engineer and pilot gave him a varied canvas of experiences and views of the world. His writing is drawn from many experiences over his 70+ years on earth and his travels to many remote parts of the planet and interaction with people. His challenge in retirement was to capture some of those experiences and make them entertaining and to leave something for his grand children and the charities he supports.

By the same Author

Coming Soon

- BEBE 2 – Resolution
- The Twilighters – Road Trip (one of a series of light hearted books)
- Coffee Maidz
- Love on Assignment
- Windfarm Warrior